THE EVIDENCE-BASED PRACTICE MANUAL

FOR

NURSES

THIRD EDITION

Edited by

Jean V Craig MSc PhD RSCN RGN
Research Associate, Norwich Medical School, Faculty of Medicine and
Health Sciences, University of East Anglia, Norwich, UK

Rosalind L Smyth MA MBBS MD FMedSci
Brough Professor of Paediatric Medicine, University of Liverpool Institute of
Child Health, Alder Hey Children's NHS Foundation Trust, Liverpool, UK

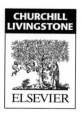

CHURCHILL
LIVINGSTONE

ELSEVIER

CHURCHILL LIVINGSTONE
ELSEVIER

© 2012 Elsevier Ltd. All rights reserved.

No part of this publication may be reproduced or transmitted in any form or by any means, electronic or mechanical, including photocopying, recording, or any information storage and retrieval system, without permission in writing from the publisher. Details on how to seek permission, further information about the Publisher's permissions policies and our arrangements with organizations such as the Copyright Clearance Center and the Copyright Licensing Agency, can be found at our website: www.elsevier.com/permissions.

This book and the individual contributions contained in it are protected under copyright by the Publisher (other than as may be noted herein).

First edition 2002
Second edition 2007
Third edition 2012

ISBN 978-0-7020-4193-8

British Library Cataloguing in Publication Data
A catalogue record for this book is available from the British Library

Library of Congress Cataloging in Publication Data
A catalog record for this book is available from the Library of Congress

Notices
Knowledge and best practice in this field are constantly changing. As new research and experience broaden our understanding, changes in research methods, professional practices, or medical treatment may become necessary.

Practitioners and researchers must always rely on their own experience and knowledge in evaluating and using any information, methods, compounds, or experiments described herein. In using such information or methods they should be mindful of their own safety and the safety of others, including parties for whom they have a professional responsibility.

With respect to any drug or pharmaceutical products identified, readers are advised to check the most current information provided (i) on procedures featured or (ii) by the manufacturer of each product to be administered, to verify the recommended dose or formula, the method and duration of administration, and contraindications. It is the responsibility of practitioners, relying on their own experience and knowledge of their patients, to make diagnoses, to determine dosages and the best treatment for each individual patient, and to take all appropriate safety precautions.

To the fullest extent of the law, neither the Publisher nor the authors, contributors, or editors, assume any liability for any injury and/or damage to persons or property as a matter of products liability, negligence or otherwise, or from any use or operation of any methods, products, instructions, or ideas contained in the material herein.

ELSEVIER your source for books, journals and multimedia in the health sciences

www.elsevierhealth.com

Working together to grow
libraries in developing countries

www.elsevier.com | www.bookaid.org | www.sabre.org

ELSEVIER   BOOK AID International   Sabre Foundation

The Publisher's policy is to use paper manufactured from sustainable forests

Printed in China

Contents

SECTION 3 THE PROCESS OF CHANGING PRACTICE

9. Using research evidence to change how services are delivered. 281
Lin Perry

10. How can we develop an evidence-based culture?. 323
Carl Thompson

Contributors

Olwen Beaven BSc(Hons) MSc
Deputy Information Specialist Manager, BMJ Evidence Centre, BMJ Group, London, UK

Bernie Carter BSc PhD PGCE PGCE RSCN SRN
Professor of Children's Nursing, Families, Children and Life Transitions Research Group, School of Nursing and Caring Sciences, University of Central Lancashire, Preston and Children's Nursing Research Unit, Alder Hey Children's NHS Foundation Trust, Liverpool, UK

Jean V Craig MSc PhD RSCN RGN
Research Associate, Norwich Medical School, Faculty of Medicine and Health Sciences, University of East Anglia, Norwich, UK

Dawn Dowding BSc(Hons) PhD RN
Professor of Applied Health Research, School of Health Care, University of Leeds, Leeds, UK

Lynne Goodacre PhD DipCOT
Honorary Lecturer, School of Health and Medicine, Lancaster University; Independent Practitioner, Preston, UK

Leanne V Jones BSc(Hons)
Research Associate, Cochrane Pregnancy and Childbirth Group, University of Liverpool, Liverpool Women's NHS Foundation Trust, Liverpool, UK

Gillian A Lancaster BSc(Hons) MSc PhD FSS CStat
Director of Postgraduate Statistics Centre and Senior Lecturer, Postgraduate Statistics Centre, Department of Mathematics and Statistics, Fylde College, Lancaster, UK

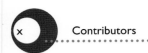

Lin Perry MSc PhD RN
Professor of Nursing Research and Practice Development,
Faculty of Nursing, Midwifery and Health, University of
Technology, Sydney, NSW, Australia

Rosalind L Smyth MA MBBS MD FMedSci
Brough Professor of Paediatric Medicine, University of
Liverpool Institute of Child Health, Alder Hey Children's NHS
Foundation Trust, Liverpool, UK

Kathleen R Stevens EdD RN ANEF FAAN
Professor and Director, Academic Center for Evidence-Based
Practice; Principal Investigator, Improvement Science Research
Network, University of Texas Health Science Center San
Antonio, San Antonio, TX, USA

Andrew C Titman BA PhD
Research Associate, Department of Mathematics and Statistics,
Fylde College, Lancaster University, Bailrigg, UK

Lois Thomas BA(Hons) PhD PGCertLTHE PGCert(Research
Degree Supervision) RN
Reader in Health Services Research, School of Nursing and
Caring Sciences, University of Central Lancashire, Preston UK

Carl Thompson PhD RN
Professor (Personal Chair), Department of Health Sciences,
University of York, York, UK

Preface

'Evidence-based' is one of the most frequently used adjectives in healthcare today. It was previously used almost exclusively in the term 'evidence-based medicine' but, happily, terms such as 'evidence-based practice' are becoming more widespread and emphasise that this is a concept that should apply to all of healthcare. Nurses, the largest group of professionals who provide healthcare, have been at the forefront in recognising the need to identify, evaluate and apply best evidence to their clinical practice. Since this manual was first published, awareness of evidence-based practice has become widespread throughout clinical practice, but professional groups can find it difficult to keep pace with the requisite knowledge and skills. This manual presents techniques for doing so in a straightforward and relevant style that will enable nurses to understand and apply evidence-based practice in their own individual settings.

As with the previous edition, the manual is divided into three sections.

Section 1 provides the background and context for evidence-based practice in nursing and gives details of some of the challenges and solutions nurses meet in ensuring that patient care is informed by scientific evidence.

Section 2 focuses on the practical skills required for identifying and interpreting research evidence to support healthcare decisions. It provides detailed, step-by-step guidance in formulating focused clinical questions, conducting successful searches of electronic databases and critically appraising a range of study designs including case control, cohort and diagnostic test accuracy studies, randomised controlled trials, qualitative research, systematic reviews and guidelines. This section culminates in a new chapter that shows how research evidence can be practically used in helping patients to reach clinical decisions.

Section 3 focuses on the strategic aspects of organizational change. The practical strategies that clinical teams and organisations need to consider if they are to promote and sustain an evaluative, evidence-based approach to their work are discussed.

All chapters in Sections 2 and 3 offer readers the opportunity to consolidate their learning by completing online exercises, for which example solutions are provided. One of the strengths of this manual has been the number of worked examples and case studies. To keep this volume relevant and contemporary, many have been replaced with new examples that illustrate how recent evidence has changed practice.

Two new chapters serve to enhance this third edition: Chapter 4 gives an overview of qualitative epistemologies, methodologies and methods and provides detailed guidance in the critical reading of qualitative research; Chapter 8 is a much-needed examination of the ways in which research evidence can be used in clinical decision-making with patients and gives practical advice on aspects such as how to communicate risks and benefits information to patients and how to use decision analysis, decision support tools and other useful techniques.

We wish our readers well as they develop and use their skills to ensure that their clinical decisions are informed by the best-available research evidence. Nurses, as a profession, are uniquely placed to understand patients' needs, priorities and beliefs and to integrate these considerations with their own expertise and with clinical evidence. The result of these endeavours is that better clinical decisions will be made and patient care will improve.

Norwich and Liverpool, 2011   Jean V Craig
Rosalind L Smyth

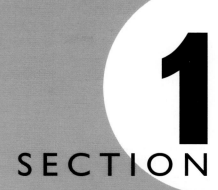

SECTION **1**

The context for evidence-based practice

CHAPTER 1

Evidence-based practice in nursing

Jean V Craig and Kathleen R Stevens

KEY POINTS

- An evidence-based approach to clinical practice aims to deliver appropriate care in an efficient manner to individual patients.

- The process entails the integration of research evidence, clinical expertise and the interpretation of patients' needs and perspectives in making decisions.

- Nursing care involves a wide range of interventions and, therefore, draws on a diverse evidence base, including, for example, evidence from psychology, sociology and public health.

- Individual nurses need to develop the key skills required to access and use evidence appropriately in clinical practice.

- Sources of synthesised evidence are evolving and are being made accessible to nurses.

- In terms of developing nurse researchers, issues such as organisational culture, management support, and career paths that accommodate both clinical and research work need to be addressed.

Evidence-based health care: what is it and why do we need it?

Evidence-based practice (EBP) has been described as 'doing the right things right' (Muir Gray 1997, p.18) so, not only doing things efficiently and to the best standard possible, but also ensuring that that which is done is of known effectiveness for that clinical situation, resulting in more good than harm. The point here is that, if we can get it right, EBP will help to improve people's experiences of illness and health care. Intuitively, few practitioners would disagree with this approach, but there are several hurdles on the way to this goal: we need the evidence base to know what it is 'right' to do (and evidence generally lags behind practice), we have to be clear to whom the evidence really applies and at what stage in their trajectory of health or illness an evidence-based intervention is indicated, and we need to implement that intervention efficiently. All this, at a time when the pressures are increasing to deliver challenging service targets and to give patients more personal choice as to how, when and where they are treated (Department of Health 2009a, 2010).

The concept of EBP is certainly not new. We would be doing our predecessors a great disservice to pretend otherwise. Let us take the example of infection control, a long-established aspect of nursing care that aims to prevent complications arising from vulnerability to infection. Semmelweis' observations on puerperal fever in the 1840s led to him insisting that doctors performing autopsies should wash their hands before going on to deliver babies, and this was associated with a marked reduction in mortality due to sepsis, from over a fifth to 3% (Rotter 1997). Similarly, it was careful observation that led John Snow in the 1840s to pinpoint a water tap in Broad Street as the cause of the outbreak of cholera in London. These examples from the 19th century encapsulate the variety of domains of professional health practice which can and should be evidence based, but they also demonstrate powerfully how reflective questioning and acutely observant practitioners can uncover evidence within their own everyday practice which, when acted upon, can improve health, although not all examples will be quite so dramatic!

It is perhaps cruelly ironic given the examples above that, in an era in which EBP is generally considered a key component of modern health care, patients are at continued risk of developing healthcare associated infections (HAIs). HAI prevalence among hospitalised patients has been identified as 5–10% in the USA (Klevens et al 2007) and 7.6% across the UK (National Audit Office 2009). In England, for example, eight out of 100 hospitalised patients included in the survey carried out between February and May 2006 had contracted a HAI (National Audit Office 2009). Estimated costs attributable to HAIs are considerable from both hospital and societal perspectives; mortality, increased length of hospital stay and financial costs are all implicated (Roberts et al 2010). HAIs are especially worrying in view of the risk of antibiotic-resistant infections such as methicillin-resistant *Staphylococcus aureus*.

Reasons for HAIs are multiple: patient factors (such as increased numbers of people with weakened immunity), therapeutic factors (increased availability of devices that breach normal defence mechanisms, inappropriate use of antibiotics), behavioural factors (inadequate hygiene practices by staff) and organisational factors (such as increased movement of patients) are all cited (Department of Health 2003a). Disappointingly, a recent scoping review of the research literature to identify effective organisational and management factors in controlling infection in general hospital settings (Griffiths et al 2009) yielded scant high-quality evidence. However, certain prerequisites for infection control were suggested: good clinical leadership; a visible presence by senior staff; a supportive environment for professional development; team stability; clearly defined responsibilities; and targeted interventions to protect patients at times of high patient turnover, high bed occupancy and/or low staffing levels. We may never win the war on HAIs, but implementing practices that are informed by evidence – where available – can help to win some of the battles.

The evidence-based movement across health care

In the early years of the evidence-based 'movement', the discourse was limited to 'medicine', rather than health care (Sackett et al 1997), but the principles of evidence-based medicine have subsequently been applied to other spheres of professional practice in health and social care such as pharmacy (Tully & Cantrill 1999), the therapies (Bury & Mead 1998), and orthodontics (Harrison 2000). Nursing has fully embraced EBP as a strategy for providing the highest quality of care (DiCenso et al. 1998, Stevens et al 2009).

The first textbook on evidence-based medicine (EBM) defined it as: 'the conscientious, explicit and judicious use of current best evidence in making decisions about the health care of patients' (Sackett et al 1997, p.2). The authors elaborated that the practice of EBM entailed the integration of individual clinical expertise with the best available external clinical evidence from systematic research, and involved taking account of the patient's perspective in making clinical decisions. Contrary to the assertions of its critics, therefore, that EBM was narrowly concerned with the conduct of randomised controlled trials and the implementation of their results in routine practice (Grahame Smith 1998), the product champions of EBM never argued that it was 'simply' a matter of slavishly following rigid guidelines based solely on the findings of trials; the need to tailor care on the basis of research evidence and clinical experience to the needs of patients was always acknowledged.

In 2000, Sackett and colleagues included the value of clinical expertise and patient perspectives more explicitly in their definition of EBM as 'the integration of best research evidence with clinical expertise and patient values' (Sackett et al 2000, p.1).

They define their terms carefully.

- **Best research evidence is defined as:**

clinically relevant research, often from the basic sciences of medicine (sic), but especially from patient-centred clinical research ... (Sackett et al 2000, p.1)

They go on to assert that:

New evidence from clinical research both invalidates previously accepted diagnostic tests and treatments and replaces them with new ones that are more powerful, more accurate, more efficacious and safer. (Sackett et al 2000, p.1)

Note that the discourse is about 'diagnostic tests' and 'treatments', whereas the broader concept of 'care' which embodies nursing practice in all settings involves much more: communication and observation, for example. This means that, in applying these principles to the variety of nursing practice, we need to draw on a range of evidence bases including from psychology and sociology.

• **Clinical expertise is defined as:**

the ability to use our clinical skills and past experience to rapidly identify each patient's unique health state and diagnosis, their individual risks and benefits of potential interventions, and their personal values and expectations. (Sackett et al 2000, p.1)

Personal professional experience, clinical judgement and even intuition have a role to play.

• **By 'patient values', the authors mean:**

the unique preferences, concerns and expectations each patient brings to a clinical encounter and which must be integrated into clinical decisions if they are to serve the patient. (Sackett et al 2000, p.1)

In reality, then, EBM is manifest by the integration of systematically derived research-based knowledge with the practitioner's tacit knowledge drawn from experience and their interpretation of the needs and perspectives of each person with whom they interact in individual clinical encounters.

The principles enunciated by Sackett and colleagues are clearly of direct relevance to all professional practice, but for any practitioner this is a daunting agenda. In the early days of EBP, we believed it meant that each individual clinician should access, appraise and synthesise evidence from primary research studies to develop EBP guidelines. Today, the move is towards research knowledge being transformed into clinical recommendations by expert panels, and embedded into healthcare delivery systems (Stevens, et al 2009) in the form of, for example, electronic prompts or reminders. That said, it remains imperative that practitioners learn to be wise users of the different types and forms of evidence integral to good patient care and to know which evidence is informative in selecting actions that have the highest likelihood of producing the intended patient outcome.

In 2000, the Institute of Medicine (IOM) published *To Err Is Human* which reported the prevalence of deaths and injury occurring from healthcare errors (IOM 2000). As a result of this publication, attention to quality and safety peaked and other widespread defects in the US healthcare system were also identified (IOM 2001). Quickly following these reports, recommendations were made in the *Quality Chasm* series that underscored the centrality of EBP as a solution in redesigning care that is effective and safe (IOM 2001, 2003, 2008). The EBP movement was significantly accelerated by these reports and key recommendations were made: i) to provide services based on scientific knowledge to all who could benefit (IOM 2001), ii) to educate all healthcare professionals to deliver evidence-based care (IOM 2003) and iii) to assess effectiveness of clinical services to provide unbiased information about what really works in health care (IOM 2008). Nurse experts echoed these recommendations: employing EBP was a competency expected of nurses (Stevens & Staley 2006) and all healthcare professionals.

In the UK, following a review of the National Health Service (NHS) led by health minister and surgeon Lord Darzi, there was a shift in health policy: whereas the emphasis had been on reducing waiting times, ensuring faster access to care and giving more choice to patients, a broader view on quality – defined as patient safety, patient experience and effectiveness of care – dictated policy (Department of Health 2008). Alongside key initiatives such as the introduction of comparable quality indicators and the publishing of patient reported/clinical outcomes to allow practitioners to benchmark their own performance against that of others, an improved information resource was introduced to aid delivery of effective care.

NHS evidence is a web-based portal giving practitioners easy access to 'authoritative clinical and non-clinical evidence and best practice' required for effective clinical decision-making. It is considered by Lord Darzi as an essential service that allows quality to be 'stitched into the very fabric of the NHS' (Department of Health 2009b). The code of conduct for nurses and midwives, implemented in May 2008, served to further embed this notion of evidence driving quality, through statements such as:

- 'You must deliver care based on the best available evidence or best practice'
- 'You must ensure any advice you give is evidence based if you are suggesting healthcare products or services'
- 'You must ensure that the use of complementary or alternative therapies is safe and in the best interests of those in your care'

(Nursing and Midwifery Council 2008).

A wide range of evidence bases relevant to nursing practice

In making decisions about therapies, investigations, service provision, etc., nurses need to draw on a wide range of evidence sources within and beyond the 'medical' sciences as illustrated by our earlier discussion of healthcare associated infections and by the examples below.

- Concordance with drug therapy can be influenced by factors ranging from unpleasant side effects of the drug, denial of illness or its significance (Beers & Berkow 1999), scepticism as to the need for the medication (Mahler et al 2010), or presence of depression or cognitive impairment (Osterberg & Blaschke

2005). The approach to the problem of poor concordance with treatment therefore requires knowledge from the psychosocial and pharmacological domains.

- Nurses wanting to introduce costly services such as a new clinic or nursing post will increasingly be obliged to present to the management team evidence on not only the effectiveness and potential harms of the intervention, but also cost-effectiveness.

- In management sciences, the research task is often to understand the organisation and how change is perceived, as much as to study the effectiveness of a complex process of change, and nurses can draw on a wide range of quantitative and qualitative research to help them become more effective managers. In the UK, a national NHS R&D programme on Service Delivery and Organisation (SDO) has been set up to increase organisational and management research in the health sector. Within this programme a stream of funding has been made available to support SDO research into nursing, midwifery and health-visiting services (www.sdo.lshtm.ac.uk/nursingandmid-wifery.htm).

- For effective communication with communities, clients and patients, nurses can draw on communication studies and psychology. Psychological research has shown that on receiving bad news, recipients retain only a limited amount of information from the first conversation; nurses can use these findings when imparting bad news, by keeping their first message simple, and providing ongoing support and repeated conversations to enable information to be given at a pace with which recipients can cope.

- Nurses working in public health roles, including health visiting, may be in a key position to advocate initiatives supported by evidence from research in the public health domain. Perhaps the best public health example is the introduction of legislation to make the wearing of seatbelts compulsory, based on epidemiological evidence of reductions in mortality. The UK Economic and Social Research Council has invested in a network of research centres that pull together the evidence base for public policy and its implementation.

Challenges

The challenge, then, for clinical nursing practice is to develop and draw on the well-focused evidence base relating to specific clinical treatments to improve the quality of clinical procedures, whilst also drawing on a more diverse evidence base for the wider concept of care which nurses provide (Pursey et al 1997). This challenge is not straightforward and there are several imperatives to be addressed.

First, the relevant research-based evidence bases are not comprehensive: there are yawning gaps in the robust evidence for much of what nurses do in the course of their daily work. Historically, academic and clinical nursing have existed as two separate entities, resulting in much research being unrelated to the 'reality' of everyday nursing practice (Pearson 2000). This historical trend in research, of prioritising professional issues over patient care issues, has had important ramifications for nurses trying to make informed decisions about aspects of clinical care, particularly with the current and long overdue emphasis given to the patient experience. The priority is to generate the evidence required, but that takes time if it is to be done properly. So what should be done when research evidence is lacking?

It is important that the recognition of the need for EBP does not result in a misguided and undiscerning dash to seek out *any* 'knowledge' available, irrespective of the quality of research on which it is based. Critical appraisal skills are crucial to enable practitioners thirsty for knowledge to discriminate between high- and low-quality evidence: to be cognisant of the strengths and weaknesses of the various research methodologies used to generate different kinds of evidence, to assess for rigour of the study design and conduct, and to be clear about to whom the research applies. Where there is no robust evidence base, the ethos of EBP should stop us in our tracks to reflect on the impact of what we are doing in the name of health, and why. Reflective practice is a key component of evidence-based health care; the very ethos of good professional practice is to reflect on the taken-for-granted assumptions that underpin everyday practice, and to routinely assess the impact and outcomes of interactions and interventions with patients, clients and the public. And we need to do all this without becoming 'frozen' and disempowered by a paucity of robust evidence.

Second, the relevant evidence bases are not static. In those areas of health care where there has been a great deal of research, it is almost impossible for any busy practitioner to keep abreast of the burgeoning body of information that emerges daily. The challenge is for information to be managed such that busy practitioners can find it accessible and be alert to its quality. We need further advances in the development of effective means by which emerging, robust evidence is integrated with the existing knowledge base in a timely manner, and made available to practitioners at time of need in a readily accessible format.

The results and conclusions of one study need to be considered in the light of other similar studies as they may differ markedly, depending on the nature of the study design and sample. An oft-quoted example is that of corticosteroids given to women expected to deliver prematurely. A number of trials did not identify clear-cut benefits of the treatment; however, when data from all trials included in a systematic review were combined in a meta-analysis (as explained in Chapter 6, page 198), it became clear that corticosteroids are effective in reducing the risk of death in babies born prematurely (Mulrow 1995). Today, systematic reviews are widely endorsed as an authoritative basis for informing practice decisions (IOM 2008).

Before a practice change is initiated, research findings need to be examined in the context of the wider evidence base. Consider, for example, the management of gastro-oesophageal reflux, a condition in which recurrent vomiting, failure to thrive, feeding difficulties and abdominal pain may be present. Infants who are placed in the prone or left lateral position have been shown to experience significantly improved outcomes (measured using the 'reflux index') compared with infants nursed on their backs (Kumar & Sarvanathan 2004); however, there is a wider body of evidence that prone or left lateral positioning in infants is a risk factor for sudden infant death syndrome

(Kumar & Sarvanathan 2004). Such evidence needs to be taken into consideration if parents are to be offered sensible, safe advice. Clinical problems need to be examined from various perspectives. If an emphasis is placed solely on determining the effectiveness of an intervention on say one narrow outcome, an oversimplified and unbalanced decision may be reached. Consideration of evidence that investigates a broader range of outcomes and patients' past experiences of the intervention could well lead to a different, more informed decision. It is hardly surprising that accessibility to just the right information (no less, no more) is flagged by nurses as an important facilitator for the adoption of an evidence-based approach to health care, as is a supportive organisational culture and opportunities for learning (Brown et al 2008).

Third, research findings should not always be transferred directly into the clinical setting: it is crucial that evidence from studies undertaken with a specific population is not inappropriately extrapolated to other population subgroups. Consider the example of evidence derived from a particular age group. The majority of clinical trials are undertaken in samples of people under the age of 65. Clinical trials in people over 80 years of age are extremely scarce (Le Quintrec et al 2005). Care should be taken, therefore, in extrapolating that evidence to older people who could have several co-existing conditions, as it will of necessity have been generated in people with few co-morbidities and that could 'confuse' the results. Randomised controlled trials have shown that thrombolytic therapy significantly reduces the risk of death in patients with acute myocardial infarction (Fibrinolytic Therapy Trialists 1994), but only 10% of the sample populations in the trials were over 74 years of age. When the results for these older participants were examined, the efficacy of the therapy was found to be ambiguous.

Healthcare organisations and individuals are responsible for ascertaining whether or not evidence is likely to be generalisable to their patient populations, thus allowing them to adapt or localise practice recommendations before piloting then implementing them and then evaluating their effect (Sigma Theta Tau 2008).

Frameworks for evidence-based practice

The most elemental concept in engaging practitioners in EBP is the *form* of knowledge (evidence) to which they connect. Knowledge should be presented in a form that has high utility to clinical decision-making. Rather than requiring practitioners to master the technical expertise to critique scientific adequacy of a primary research study, their point-of-care decisions would be much better supported with recommendations that have been based on all existing research knowledge and vetted by clinical experts.

The ACE Star Model of Knowledge Transformation (Stevens 2004) provides a framework with which to consider the transformation of knowledge from its point of discovery to its impact on patient and healthcare outcomes. Depicted as a five-point star to indicate the various stages of knowledge transformation, the Model is conceptualized as follows. (1) Discovery: undertaking a primary research study such as a survey, a randomised controlled trial or qualitative enquiry. (2) Evidence summary: synthesising the evidence from primary research studies, ideally using rigorous systematic review methodology. (3) Translation: developing EBP guidelines; a process in which experts consider the evidential base, combine it with expertise and theory and extend recommendations for practice. (4) Integration: practice is aligned or realigned to reflect best evidence and is tailored to the particular healthcare setting and patient-centred preferences. (5) Evaluation: taking an inclusive view of the impact that the EBP has on patient health outcomes, satisfaction, efficacy and efficiency of care and health policy. Quality improvement of healthcare processes and outcomes is the goal of knowledge transformation. A preferred starting point in moving evidence into clinical decisions is point 3: finding clinical recommendations that are clearly evidence based. Once this is accomplished, the clinician considers point 4, integration into practice, and adopts the recommendations into local practice.

Other models for EBP include the Iowa Model (Titler et al. 2001) which targets clinical guidelines and the social system into which the guidelines are adopted, and the Joanna Briggs Institute (JBI) Model in which clinical decision-making is a pivotal point of best evidence, context, client preference and professional judgement (Pearson et al 2005). The four major components of this model are recognised as evidence generation, evidence synthesis, evidence transfer, and evidence utilisation.

Models can contribute to our understanding of how to change practice in the light of best evidence often within the context of knowledge translation/translational science. Although models often contain overlapping concepts, they may offer differing but important perspectives on how to achieve an evidence-based approach to care (Mitchell & Fisher, in press). Part of the scientific work needed in the field is the continued development of theoretical frameworks to guide the process.

Workforce competencies for evidence-based practice

The new competencies that emerged with the EBP movement require healthcare professionals to engage in knowledge (evidence) management—to access knowledge, to appraise knowledge, and to integrate new knowledge into practice changes. Continued professional development for life-long learning has long been recognized as essential to quality care (Department of Health 2001, IOM 2001) and, in the past decade, EBP competencies have been articulated across health professions (IOM 2003).

Specifically in nursing, EBP competencies were developed from several perspectives. In the US, following the recommendations that each health profession must develop its specific competencies, national consensus was established across a set of 82 competency statements; the competencies were organised around the five ACE Star Model Points (discovery, summary, translation, integration, and evaluation) and across three levels of professional preparation (basic, intermediate and advanced). These competencies guide the retooling of current workforce as well as the preparation (education) of future workforce. They form the foundation for the ACE Evidence-Based Practice Readiness Inventory, a survey of self-efficacy in employing EBP (Stevens 2009).

Because a requisite of knowledge management is *access* to that knowledge, another approach assessed nurses' ability to access and use computers to locate evidence (Pravikoff et al 2005). This assessment focused only on the tools and skills to obtain evidence, so informed a more limited set of competencies.

Following these developments, a wide-spread effort emerged to support the identification of competencies for quality and safety education in nursing (Cronenwett et al 2007). Within this ongoing project, national panels are engaged in identifying competencies in EBP, patient-centred care, teamwork and collaboration, quality improvement, safety and informatics, reflecting the recommendations from IOM (2003). To assist with the full adoption into educational programmes, the Quality and Safety Education for Nurses programme includes significant teaching-learning resources on the website (QSEN 2010). Specific EBP competencies are now included as essential competencies for baccalaureate, masters, and doctoral education in the United States (AACN 2010).

Nursing education has undergone transformation in response to the EBP movement. The current workforce, new workforce, and future workforce are essential in successfully shifting the paradigm of care to fully employing EBP. Education, professional development, and performance expectations are powerful factors in achieving this change.

Welcome developments

We have demonstrated that the concept of EBP is not new, but it is reassuring that the commitment to the concept is so firmly stated in policies. (Australian Government Department of Health and Ageing 2006, Department of Health 2006, IOM 2008, National Institutes of Health 2005). In the UK, the strategy for nursing, *Making a Difference*, reflects this commitment and emphasises the need for a robust evidence base for nursing, midwifery and health visiting (Department of Health 1999). The vision for nursing in the 21st century is for all nurses to seek out evidence and apply it in their everyday practice, with an increasing proportion actively participating in research and development, and some developing into research leaders (Department of Health 2006). But to what extent have we ensured that vibrant R&D activity around nursing issues and perspectives (whether or not it is undertaken by nurses) is really embedded in nursing practice, and that the results are implemented?

A number of strategies have been implemented and some are starting to pay dividends. For example, nursing (or practice) development units (NDU) were set up as 'hot-houses for innovation and change in nursing practice' (Redfern et al 1997). The staff of these units are ideally placed to take a leading role in establishing EBP for nursing; in addition, several of the units have been awarded research grants. Urinary catheterisation is just one topic that has been explored in the light of Sackett and colleagues' (1997) definition of EBP and the organisational infrastructure required for achieving desired outcomes (Adams & Cooke 1998).

The benchmarking process outlined in *The Essence of Care* (Department of Health 2003b) is another development that has the potential to increase an evidence-based approach to nursing care. Different types of evidence have been used to establish benchmark standards which can be used as a starting point for comparing practice, identifying optimum practice and seeking methods to remedy poor practice. To illustrate, following the launch of the paediatric continence services benchmark in 2001, a participating organisation identified a number of shortfalls in their service: inconsistencies in provision of care across the district; poorly defined patient pathways and discrepancies in information giving. Subsequent collaboration with a neighbouring healthcare provider with an excellent paediatric continence service is now underway and aims to improve referral routes, integrate the service across all sectors and develop training programmes that facilitate an evidence-based approach to care (NHS Modernisation Agency 2004).

In terms of developing a cadre of nurse researchers, there have been key issues concerning the availability of career paths that enable a combination of research and everyday practice, organisational culture and management support for the research ethos in clinical areas, and colleagues' disdain for or downright jealousy about the research role as they witness it. For example, the potential profile of nurses' involvement in R&D has not been enhanced by the experience of some research nurses: employed on short-term contracts, collecting data for medical colleagues in clinical trials, and without any tangible development of personal research potential or acknowledgement in publications (Department of Health 1999). Thankfully, clinical researcher career paths for nurses are now finally a reality, reflected in the availability of clinical academic training fellowships such as those offered by the UK National Institute of Health Research. It can be found at (http://www.nihrtcc.nhs.uk/cat/).

The healthcare research strategy within the UK is undergoing a fundamental revision in recognition of the role that research can play in improving the health and well-being of the population. The overall aims are for the system to be more responsive to the research needs of patients, the public, healthcare professionals and policy makers; for world-class support to be available to researchers; and for healthcare organisations to develop the infrastructure required for high-quality research (Department of Health 2006). Research in all healthcare areas, including prevention of ill health, promotion of health, disease management, patient care, delivery of health care and its organisation, public health and social care, is included in the strategy.

The welcome commitment to leadership and R&D within the nursing, midwifery and health-visiting professions surely presents us with a golden opportunity. We now need to get on with it, and work to ensure that the next generation of nurses, and those from previous generations who stay (or return), take it for granted that they should seek out and appraise research findings and apply them. This is not always easy, but we owe it to the public to apply our imagination and enthusiasm to make sure that the care they receive is based on the best available evidence.

REFERENCES

Adams, F., Cooke, M., 1998. Implementing evidence-based practice for urinary catheterisation. Br. J. Nurs. 7 (22), 1393–1399.

American Association of Colleges of Nursing (AACN), 2010. AACN "Essentials" Series. Available http://www.aacn.nche.edu/Education/essentials.htm (accessed 30.09.10.).

Australian Government Department of Health and Ageing, 2006. Australian Better Health Initiative. Available online at: www.health.gov.au/internet/wcms/publishing.nsf (accessed February 2006).

Beers, M.H., Berkow, R. (Eds.), 1999. Factors affecting drug response. In: Merck manual of diagnosis and therapy, seventeenth ed. Merck Research Laboratories, New Jersey.

Brown, C.E., Wickline, M.A., Ecoff, L., Glaser, D., 2008. Knowledge, attitudes and perceived barriers to evidence-based practice at an academic medical center. J. Adv. Nurs. 65 (2), 371–381.

Bury, T.J., Mead, J.M. (Eds.), 1998. Evidence-based healthcare: a practical guide for therapists. Butterworth-Heinemann, Oxford.

Cronenwett, L., Sherwood, G., Barnsteiner, J., Disch, J., Johnson, J., Mitchell, P., et al., 2007. Quality and safety education for nurses. Nurs. Outlook 55 (3), 122–131.

Department of Health, 1999. Making a difference: strengthening the nursing, midwifery and health visiting contribution to health and health care. Department of Health, London.

Department of Health, 2001. Working together – learning together: a framework for lifelong learning for the NHS. Department of Health, London.

Department of Health, 2003a. Winning ways. Working together to reduce healthcare associated infection in England. Department of Health, London.

Department of Health/NHS Modernisation Agency, 2003b. The essence of care. Patient-focused benchmarks for clinical governance. Department of Health, London.

Department of Health, 2006. Best research for best health. A new national research health strateg. Department of Health, London.

Department of Health, 2008. High quality care for all: NHS next stage review final report. Department of Health, London.

Department of Health, 2009a. Implementation of the right to choice and information set out in the NHS Constitution. Department of Health, London.

Department of Health, 2009b. High quality care for all: our journey so far. Department of Health, London.

Department of Health, 2010. Improving the health and well-being of people with long term conditions. Department of Health, London.

DiCenso, A., Cullum, N., Ciliska, D., 1998. Implementing evidence based nursing: some misconceptions (editorial). Evid. Based Nurs. 1, 38–40.

Fibrinolytic Therapy Trialists (FTT) Collaborative Group, 1994. Indications for fibrinolytic therapy in suspected acute myocardial infarction: collaborative overview of early mortality and major morbidity results from all randomised trials of over 1000 patients. Lancet 343, 311–322.

Grahame Smith, D., 1998. Evidence based medicine: challenging the authority. J. R. Soc. Med. 35 (Suppl.), 7–11.

Griffiths, P., Renz, A., Hughes, J., Rafferty, A.M., 2009. Impact of organisation and management factors on infection control in hospitals: a scoping review. American Journal of Hospital Infections 73 (1), 1–14.

Harrison, J.E., 2000. Evidence-based orthodontics – how do I assess the evidence? J. Orthod. 27 (2), 189–197.

Institute of Medicine, 2000. To err is human: building a safer health system. National Academies Press, Washington, DC.

Institute of Medicine, 2001. Crossing the quality chasm: a new health system for the 21st century. National Academies Press, Washington, DC.

Institute of Medicine, 2003. Health professions education: a bridge to quality. National Academies Press, Washington, DC.

Institute of Medicine, 2008. Knowing what works in healthcare: a roadmap for the nation. National Academies Press, Washington, DC.

Klevens, R.M., Edwards, J.R., Richards, C.L., et al., 2007. Estimating health care-associated infections and deaths in US hospitals in 2002. Public Health Rep. 122, 160–166.

Kumar, Y., Sarvanathan, R., 2004. Gastro-oesophageal reflux in children. Clin. Evid. Available online at: www.clinicalevidence.com.

Le Quintrec, J.L., Bussy, C., Golmard, J.L., Hervé, C., Baulon, A., Piette, F., 2005. Randomized controlled drug trials on very elderly subjects: descriptive and methodological analysis of trials published between 1990 and 2002 and comparison with trials on adults. J. Gerontol. A Biol. Sci. Med. Sci. 60, 340–344.

Mahler, C., Hermann, K., Horne, R., Jank, S., Haefeli, W.E., Szecsenyi, J., 2010. Patients' beliefs about medicines in a primary care setting in Germany. J. Eval. Clin. Pract. Nov 18. doi:10.1111/j.1365-2753.2010.01589.x. [Epub ahead of print].

Mitchell, S.A., Fisher, C., In press. Theoretical pluralism to advance evidence-based practice and translational science in nursing. Nurs. Outlook.

Muir Gray, J.A., 1997. Evidence-based health care: how to make health policy and management decisions. Churchill Livingstone, New York.

Mulrow, C.D., 1995. Rationale for systematic reviews. In: Chalmers, I., Altman, D.G. (Eds.), Systematic reviews. BMJ Publishing Group, London.

National Audit Office Report by the Controller and Auditor General, 2009. Reducing healthcare associated infections in hospitals in England. Report: HC 560 Session 2008-2009. http://www.nao.org. uk/publications/0809/reducing_healthcare_associated.aspx.

National Institutes of Health, US Department of Health and Human Services, 2005. About NIH, Available online at: www.nih.gov/ about (accessed January 2006).

NHS Modernisation Agency, 2004. Good practice in paediatric continence services – benchmarking in action. Available online at: www.cgsupport.nhs.uk/PDFs/articles/good_practice_paediatric_ continence_services.pdf. November 2010.

Nursing and Midwifery Council, 2008. The code: Standards of conduct, performance and ethics for nurses and midwives. http://www.nmc-uk.org/Nurses-and-midwives/The-code/ The-code-in-full/ (accessed 04.12.10).

Osterberg, L., Blaschke, T., 2005. Adherence to medication. N. Engl. J. Med. 353, 487–497.

Pearson, M., 2000. Making a difference through research: how nurses can turn the vision into reality (editorial). NT Research 5 (2), 85–86.

Pearson, A., Wiechula, R., Court, A., Lockwood, C., 2005. The JBI model of evidence-based healthcare. International Journal of Evidence-Based Healthcare 8 (3), 207–215.

Pravikoff, D.S., Tanner, A.B., Pierce, S.T., 2005. Readiness of U.S. nurses for evidence-based practice. Am. J. Nurs. 9 (105), 40–51.

Pursey, A., Quinney, D., Pearson, M., 1997. Concepts of care in primary health care nursing. In: Hugman, R., Peelo, M., Soothill, K. (Eds.), Concepts of care. Edward Arnold, London.

Quality and Safety Education for Nurses (QSEN), 2010. About QSEN. Available http://www.qsen.org/about_qsen.php (accessed 2.10.10).

Redfern, S., Norman, I., Murrells, T., et al., 1997. External review of the Department of Health-funded nursing development units. Executive Summary. Available from Nursing Research Unit, King's College London, Cornwall House, Waterloo Road, London SE1 8WA.

Roberts, R.R., Scott, 2nd, R.D., Hota, B., et al., 2010. Costs attributable to healthcare-acquired infection in hospitalized adults and a comparison of economic methods. Med. Care 48 (11), 1026–1035.

Rotter, M.L., 1997. 150 years of hand disinfection. Semmelweis' heritage. Hygiene und Medizin 22, 332–339.

Sackett, D., Richardson, W.S., Rosenberg, W., Haynes, R.B., 1997. Evidence based medicine: how to practice and teach EBM. Churchill Livingstone, New York.

Sackett, D., Strauss, S.E., Richardson, W.S., Rosenberg, W., Haynes, R.B., 2000. Evidence-based medicine. How to practise and teach EBM, second ed. Churchill Livingstone, London.

Sigma Theta Tau International 2005–2007 Research and Scholarship Advisory Committee, 2008. International position status on evidence-based practice. Worldviews Evid. Based Nurs. Second Quarter, 57–59.

Stevens, K.R., 2004. ACE Star Model of EBP: knowledge transformation. Academic Center for Evidence-based Practice. The University of Texas Health Science Center, San Antonio. www.acestar.uthscsa.edu.

Stevens, K.R., Staley, J., 2006. The quality chasm reports, evidence-based practice, and nursing's response to improve healthcare. Nurs. Outlook 54 (2), 94–101.

Stevens, K.R., 2009. Essential competencies for evidence-based practice in nursing, second ed. Academic Center for Evidence-based Practice (ACE) of University of Texas Health Science Center, San Antonio.

Stevens, K.R., McDuffie, K., Clutter, P.C., 2009. Research and the mandate for evidence-based practice, quality, and safety. In: Mateo, M., Kirchhoff, K. (Eds.), Research for advance practice nurses: from evidence to practice. Springer Publishing Company, New York, pp. 43–70.

Titler, M., Kleiber, C., Steelman, V., et al., 2001. The iowa model of evidence-based practice to promote quality care. Critical Care Clinics of North America 13 (4), 497–509.

Tully, M.P., Cantrill, J., 1999. Role of the pharmacist in evidence-based prescribing in primary care. In: Gabbay, M. (Ed.), The evidence-based primary care handbook. Royal Society of Medicine, London, pp. 183–193.

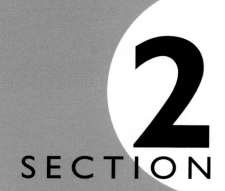

SECTION 2

Skills for evidence-based practice

CHAPTER 2

How to ask the right question

Jean V Craig

KEY POINTS

- Clinical decisions should take account of best available current research evidence.

- The process of achieving this usually requires a number of steps: recognising a need for information, seeking out research evidence to address that need, assessing the validity of that evidence, ascertaining what the results mean and deciding whether the results are applicable for a particular clinical circumstance.

- A starting point of this process entails turning a need for information into a precise, carefully thought-through question that can drive and shape each step.

- A well-formulated question provides the key to efficient and effective searching for research evidence. It maximises the potential for finding relevant evidence that can be applied to a specific patient in a specific setting.

- 'PICO' provides a useful framework to prompt consideration of each component of a question and is a helpful way of thinking through clinical problems.

- In effect, the PICO framework encourages careful thought as to the features of research studies that may be useful in informing specific clinical decisions.

Introduction

The process for ensuring that clinical decisions are, as far as possible, informed by current research evidence has been described by Sackett et al (2000). This approach entails:

1. converting information needs about clinical problems into clear questions

2. seeking evidence to answer those questions

3. evaluating (critically appraising) the evidence for its validity (truthfulness) and usefulness

4. integrating findings with clinical expertise, patient needs and patient preferences to reach a decision as to the optimum course of action, and then applying this decision

5. evaluating performance (and the outcome of the decision).

This approach is driven by the belief that up-to-date, well-conducted research, when used judiciously to inform clinical decisions, can help to improve patients' outcomes.

An important first step of the process is to clarify what information is needed to inform a particular aspect of nursing care, and to translate that information need into an explicit and succinct question that will drive the subsequent steps of the process. A carefully formulated question maximises the likelihood that relevant, high-quality evidence is identified and incorporated appropriately into the decision-making process. Where questions are poorly defined or where a haphazard approach is used to find papers, the likely result is hours of non-focused reading of literature that may or may not be relevant or applicable to the topic of interest. Developing 'answerable' clinical questions is thus an invaluable skill for nurses aiming to integrate best research evidence with other key elements of decision-making (such as clinical expertise, patient preferences and values, resource availability) when caring for patients.

This chapter describes how to frame questions for interrogating the research evidence. It presents one example of a standardised format for question formulation (as suggested by Sackett et al 1997), and uses clinical examples to illustrate its use.

Information for effective nursing care

Nurses, along with other healthcare practitioners, are required to make numerous decisions when caring for their patients. Consider the following examples of nursing care/interventions carried out during the course of a morning by a nurse working in a general practice:

- Syringing the ears of an elderly gentleman complaining of increasing deafness due to wax build-up
- Discussing asthma preventative measures with a teenager who has frequent episodes of asthma
- Performing a cervical smear test
- Advising a young man on interventions to alleviate acute lower back pain
- Running a clinic for patients with type 2 diabetes mellitus.

The information that the nurse needs for managing each of these clinical episodes is extensive and varied. To successfully care for the patient presenting with wax build-up in his ears, the nurse might need an understanding of the purpose of ear wax and of the anatomy of the external auditory canal and tympanic membrane (think of these as foundational or background information needs), as well as knowledge of the effectiveness and comparative benefits and harms of each of the available interventions, and how well they are tolerated by patients (think of these as more specific, foreground information needs). Foundational (background) information, whilst not static, does not always change rapidly, so textbooks might be a suitable resource for accessing such information. In contrast, foreground information is best obtained from up-to-date research articles. The starting point for successfully tracking down such research articles is the focused 'answerable' question. Before looking at methods for focusing questions, briefly consider some of the foreground information that our practice nurse might need when caring for his or her patients. Examples are presented in Box 2.1.

Let's consider the available research evidence for the first question in Box 2.1: 'Which method should I use to remove ear wax?' Water, olive oil, cerumol, sodium bicarbonate, glycerine, saline, acetic acid and docusate sodium are just some of the liquids or ear drops used for the purpose of softening ear wax and may be used in combination with mechanical methods of wax removal such as ear irrigation, in which a syringe is used to wash wax out of the ear canal, ear curettes, forceps or micro-suction (Burton & Doree 2003, Clegg et al 2010). Patients that

---

BOX 2.1 Examples of information needed

- Which method should I use to remove ear wax?
- What reasons do teenagers give for avoiding taking preventative asthma medication?
- How can I persuade this patient to take his asthma treatments regularly?
- Why does this patient have so many asthma attacks?
- What is the best method of delivering the asthma drugs?
- Do cervical smear tests with normal results accurately exclude cervical cancer?
- Should I test for chlamydia at the time of cervical smear?
- What advice should I give to this young man with back pain?
- What is the best way of monitoring for complications of diabetes?
- What is the most effective way of helping patients with diabetes to increase their level of physical activity?

self-treat may use wax softeners, cotton buds (with the attendant risks of damage to the external ear canal) and soft bulb irrigators (only recently available). There are reports from the early 1990s of harm occurring with ear irrigation. Damage to the external auditory canal, infection, perforation of the tympanic membrane, pain and vertigo have all been reported (Dinsdale et al 1991, Sharp et al 1990, Zikk et al 1991, Zivik & King 1993). In a review conducted by the Medical Defence Union (MDU), ear syringing was shown to account for 19% of claims involving general practice procedures, and in more than half of the claims it was the practice nurse who performed the procedure (Price 1997). Complications appeared to be related to poor technique, faulty equipment, exertion of excess pressure and failure to examine the ear (Price 1997). Modern, electronic pulsed syringes have now largely replaced the old-fashioned metal syringes, for which the rate of irrigation had to be manually controlled. Given the potential for excessive pressure to be exerted on the plunger of the metal syringes, the risk of ear injury was greater with these devices. Despite the availability of electronic pulsed syringes, ear irrigation is contraindicated in people with previous tympanic membrane perforation, grommets, mastoid surgery or chronic middle ear disease and in patients where the ear in question is the person's only hearing ear.

A systematic review of studies investigating different methods of wax removal found limited good-quality evidence to guide clinical decisions with regard to adverse events, cost-effectiveness, wax clearance, improved quality of life and satisfaction (Clegg et al 2010). Softeners were reported to have an effect in clearing wax when used alone or as a precursor to irrigation, but evidence as to which softeners are the most effective was reported to be inconclusive. Evidence on the effectiveness of mechanical removal of wax was limited and was reported to be equivocal. Adverse events from wax softeners were reported to be rare and mild in nature. There were very few serious adverse events from mechanical removal of wax reported in the trials included in the systematic review, but the authors caution that this may have been due to the design of the studies included in the systematic review and too short a follow-up of patients in some of the included studies.

How does this evidence help our practice nurse? When discussing treatment options with the patient, the nurse can draw on this information to explain that it is not yet known which method of wax removal is the most effective, that wax softeners appear to be more effective than no treatment, and that ear syringing with an electronic syringe carries a slightly greater (although rare) risk of serious adverse events than wax softeners. Using this information, the nurse and patient can reach a decision that is right for the patient, taking account of the severity of the problem and its impact on the patient's quality of life.

So, the evidence is potentially useful to our practice nurse, but only if it can be tracked down. The questions listed in Box 2.1 don't really guide the search for evidence. This is because they fail to indicate the specific additional items of information that the nurse needs to solve each problem (Greenhalgh 1997). Methods for asking focused, 'answerable' questions are discussed below.

Turning information needs into focused questions

There is an art to phrasing questions in such a way as to elicit a meaningful answer, whether these are questions directed at people or questions asked of the research literature.

As with the research process, the evidence-based process flows from the question. When conducting research, the study design and methods are determined by what the researcher wants to know, i.e. by the research question. Similarly, in using research, i.e. when aiming to incorporate best evidence in clinical decision-making, it is the clinical question that drives each step of the process: it guides the search for relevant evidence, it guides the sorting of best evidence from weaker, less valid evidence, and helps to frame whether the evidence is applicable to the patients and setting in which it is to be used. We will look at this in more detail.

Searching for evidence

The more explicit the question, the easier it is to develop a search strategy to interrogate the electronic databases containing health-care publications (such as CINAHL (Cumulative Index of Allied Health and Nursing Literature), MEDLINE, EMBASE or the databases contained within the Cochrane Library). Search strategies generally aim to yield a manageable number of relevant research studies, whilst at the same time not missing too many relevant studies. The key components of the clinical question inform the search strategy. The less focused the question, the larger the numbers of non-relevant studies that will be identified, and the more time wasted by having to sift through unnecessarily long lists of references looking for relevant studies.

To illustrate, the practice nurse wants to know what advice to give to a young man with back pain (Box 2.1). If she or he searched the MEDLINE database from 2005 to 2010, using the phrase 'back pain', this would yield just over 9000 references. Even limiting the search to the most recent year would result in an unmanageable number of references (more than 1900) (search carried out 4/12/10). A quick glance at the references retrieved by this search shows us that many of the articles relate to pregnancy and childbirth, and are, therefore, unlikely to be of relevance to the male patient who presented with the complaint. A focused question would help to overcome this problem by providing guidance to the search strategy.

Selecting the best evidence

Once the question has been formulated, the type of study design that will best answer that question becomes clear (Logan & Gilbert 2000). Chapter 5 discusses study designs and their 'hierarchy' in terms of producing valid evidence for particular research questions. For the moment, it is sufficient to have a broad understanding of which study design best addresses a particular question. A question about the effectiveness of a treatment is best addressed by a well-conducted systematic review of randomised controlled trials (RCTs), or by an RCT in which participants are randomly allocated to receive or not receive an intervention, with the groups followed up for the outcome event of interest. The point of randomisation is that it avoids the possibility of selection bias (i.e. bias due to systematic differences between the groups in their prognosis or responsiveness to the treatment) (*Bandolier* 2004).

Where information about the prognosis of a disease is required, the best evidence would be provided by a good-quality cohort study. Prognosis refers to the possible outcomes of an illness, and the frequency with which these outcomes occur (Laupacis et al 1994). Patient characteristics that are strongly associated with a particular outcome are called prognostic factors. It is usually impossible (and indeed unethical) to randomise patients to different prognostic factors, and so the RCT is not an appropriate study design for investigating prognosis (Laupacis et al 1994). Instead, a cohort study is conducted where one or more groups (cohorts) who have not yet developed the specified outcome event are followed forward in time and the number of events recorded for each cohort.

A less robust study design for prognostic studies is the case-control study where participants who have already developed the specified outcome event (cases) are compared with participants who do not have the same outcomes (controls). The researchers look back in time to see what percentage of participants in each group has the prognostic factor. Case–control studies are particularly useful where the outcome is rare or where a long follow-up is required (Laupacis et al 1994). Case–control studies can also be used to investigate aetiology (the cause) of disease. Here researchers look back in time to establish the percentage of 'cases' and 'controls' that have experienced the exposure of interest.

For a question relating to a patient's understanding of their condition or perceptions of an intervention, the best evidence would be a well-conducted qualitative study, of which there are numerous approaches. Regardless of the approach, qualitative research is committed to viewing the phenomenon of interest from the perspective of the people being studied (Bryman 1988), and thus aims to give insight into the different meanings and values that people may attribute to 'events'. Further information on qualitative research is given in Chapter 4.

A search of electronic databases may yield a large number of research studies that appear to be relevant to the clinical question. Knowing which type of study design would best answer the question enables rapid sorting of the retrieved studies such that studies with the most appropriate study design take precedence. It is worth remembering that the preferred study design (summarised in Box 2.2) is not always feasible in terms of costs, time or ethical considerations, and researchers might have to resort to less than optimal study designs. Box 2.2 is certainly not comprehensive but provides a flavour of different types of questions and preferred study designs.

Applying the evidence

When a well-conducted study has been located, a judgement has to be made as to whether the results from the research would be achieved if they were applied to a specific patient in

---

BOX 2.2 Optimal study designs according to clinical question

Questions about effectiveness of an intervention
Randomised controlled trial (or systematic review thereof)

Questions about the accuracy of a diagnostic test
Studies that compare the new test against a reference standard test

Questions about prognosis
Cohort studies or, when the outcome is rare or the required duration of follow-up is long, case–control studies

Questions about aetiology (causation)
Case–control or cohort study

Questions about perceptions, attitudes, beliefs
Qualitative research (numerous approaches)

your setting. It is unlikely that the circumstances in which the research study was undertaken will exactly match your clinical situation, and this may affect the applicability or transferability of the study results. When reading a research study, it is important to decide whether the participants included in the study are so dissimilar from your patient/setting that the results cannot be applied. Is it appropriate, for example, to apply the findings of a study that looked at methods for improving adherence to drug treatment in the elderly to a population of teenagers? Methods that are effective in the elderly, such as the dispensing of tablets into individual containers labelled with the days of the week, may be seen by adolescents as embarrassing and may in fact result in reduced compliance. Similarly, a judgement must be made as to whether a similar, but not identical, intervention or test will be likely to produce the same result as that achieved in the study. As shown below, the carefully formulated question usually includes a description of the patient group of interest, the planned treatment(s) or investigation(s), and the key outcomes that the patient hopes to achieve. It is therefore a useful tool for screening out those research studies that are not applicable to the clinical situation or for helping to ensure that differences between the patient and the research population are transparent.

A framework for formulating questions

The PICO (population, intervention, comparison intervention, outcome) framework, devised by Sackett et al (1997), is a useful method for clarifying exactly what your question is. It can help you to fine-tune your question in advance of seeking out research evidence. The question is built in four (or three) parts (Box 2.3). Careful thought is required when deciding how general or specific each part of the question should be.

In terms of **population,** your goal may be to find evidence from research conducted in patients with a specific disease regardless of their age, gender, disease severity or co-morbidities. However, there may be good reasons for restricting your search

---

BOX 2.3 The four (or three)-part question (PICO)

Patient or problem:	Define who or what the question is about. *Tip: describe a group of patients similar to yours*
Intervention:	Define which intervention, test or exposure you are interested in. An intervention is a planned course of action. An exposure is something that happens such as a fall, anxiety, exposure to house dust mites, etc. (Bury & Mead 1998). *Tip: describe what it is you are considering doing or what it is that has happened to the patient*
Comparison intervention (if any):	Define the alternative intervention. *Tip: describe the alternative that can be compared with the intervention*
Outcomes:	Define the important outcomes, beneficial or harmful. *Tip: Define what you are hoping to achieve or avoid*

---

to studies undertaken in a more 'select' group of patients. This will depend on whether or not the results of studies undertaken in a very broad, inclusive research population would be generalisable to your specific patient. If, for example, there are good clinical reasons for suspecting that the results from studies conducted in hospitalised patients are unlikely to be applicable to your patient in the primary care setting, then the population part of the question should reflect this. By carefully thinking through, and recognising that your population of interest comprises patients receiving primary care, you can devise a search strategy that targets studies undertaken in this population (by incorporating search terms such as general practice or GP or family doctor). When sorting through the studies retrieved by the search you can immediately put to one side those publications that report on hospitalised patients only. Of course, such studies may provide some useful information, but if good-quality studies are available that investigate primary care patients why bother with them?

The **intervention** (or test or exposure) that you are interested in learning about and the **comparison intervention** (if any) may need to be described in some detail to ensure clarity. This is especially important for multifaceted interventions such as asthma clinics, nurse development units, etc., where any number of factors may be responsible for the outcome of interest. Describing the duration or frequency of the intervention and the method of applying the intervention may be an important factor in helping you to select studies that have investigated an intervention that best matches one that you are able to provide, but you may want to be less prescriptive here, particularly if there is scope for you to adapt your intervention to match any research-proven interventions identified in the search.

Deciding on the most important **outcomes** is not always straightforward, but can be facilitated by considering the patient's perspective alongside the perspectives of the healthcare practitioner and funder. The point here is that you want to seek out studies that have investigated important outcomes, not just studies that have investigated easy-to-measure but non-informative outcomes.

The PICO formula cannot always be easily applied, but nevertheless it is a useful tool. The Scenarios below illustrate the use of this formula.

 ## SCENARIO 2.1

A 10-year-old girl who has had open-heart surgery has been very ill for 2 days, requiring artificial ventilation and a number of support drugs to maintain her blood pressure. She has developed a small pressure sore at the back of her head.

The nurse asks the following question:
How can I prevent further pressure sores from developing in this child?

This general question may be difficult to answer. Many factors contribute to tissue breakdown, including poor nutrition, poor circulation, immobility and type of mattress. The nurse decides to focus on the mattress. The child is currently being nursed on a high-specification foam mattress.

At this stage, further defining each component of the question will yield dividends when searching for, and sorting through, relevant research studies.

Population

The nurse must decide whether research carried out in the adult population could be applied to children. The decision of whether to exclude specific age groups is usually based on the known differences in the response to disease, treatments and tests, by each age group, or on the inferred differences which might arise from the above. If the differences are such that the results of a research study will not be generalisable from one age group to another, then age groups should be defined within the question.

In addition, it is important to consider whether, and how specifically, to define the condition. Is there any reason for restricting the question to patients who have had cardiac surgery? Critically ill cardiac patients may have poor circulation and, therefore, be at increased risk of developing pressure sores; however, other groups of critically ill children (for example children with septicaemia) might also have poor perfusion. One could argue that all critically ill children are at increased risk of developing pressure sores, and research carried out in these patients, regardless of their diagnosis, would help to answer the question.

Intervention (or test or exposure)

A variety of mattresses and beds are available on the market, ranging from standard hospital foam or high-specification foam to constant low-pressure devices or alternating pressure devices. Some of these devices may be more effective than others. Depending on the device under consideration, there could be major cost implications. In the year 2000, costs of pressure-relieving devices were found to range from £100 to £30 000 (Cullum et al 2000). The nurse does not want to overly restrict the question, thereby limiting the chance of finding any relevant evidence, but by clarifying what pressure-relieving device could be used for the 10-year-old patient (we will assume this to be the constant low-pressure bed), the search for information is made easier.

Comparison intervention

It is not always necessary to define a comparison intervention, but in this case the intervention against which the proposed device could be compared is the method currently in use. In this scenario, this is the high-specification foam mattress.

Outcome

Outcomes may need to be carefully defined. The nurse wants to prevent further pressure sores, but what does she or he mean by pressure sore? The results of studies in which a pressure sore is described as 'full-thickness skin loss' might differ from those of studies that include in their definition 'persistent discolouration of the skin, or partial-thickness skin loss'. Ideally, the identified research would provide data on the outcome that is of interest to the nurse.

In summary:

- *Population*: Critically ill children
- *Intervention*: Constant low-pressure beds
- *Comparison*: High-specification foam mattresses
- *Outcome*: Pressure sores at any stage: constant discolouration of skin, or partial- or full-thickness skin loss.

Our more focused question could therefore be:
In critically ill children, are constant low-pressure beds more effective than high-specification foam mattresses in preventing

pressure sores (defined here as constant discolouration of the skin, or partial- or full-thickness skin loss)?

At this stage it is useful to identify which type of *study design* is most likely to provide a valid (believable) answer to the question. As this is a question about effectiveness of a therapy, the study design of choice is a systematic review of RCTs or a RCT (see Chapter 5 for more information). Retrieved studies can be sorted accordingly, with studies of the above design being given highest priority.

Searching for research evidence is covered in detail in Chapter 3, but it is worth briefly mentioning here that it is not always necessary or, indeed, desirable to use all four parts of the question when developing a search strategy. The nurse could run a preliminary search using terms relating to the *population* (in this case, terms such as 'child', 'paediatric', 'critically ill', etc.) and *intervention* ('low-pressure bed', etc.) parts of the question. If this resulted in an unmanageable number of references, terms relating to the *comparison intervention* or even the *outcome* could also be added, but with caution, as explained in Chapter 3. (Searching on all four components of the question will restrict the number of references identified and will enhance the likelihood of these references being relevant to the question BUT will also risk relevant articles not being identified.) A filter could be added to the search so that only studies of a particular design are retrieved. Search filters are discussed in Chapter 3.

The nurse will be able to check the retrieved articles against the focused question. Those that are found to be less applicable (for example, studies that have focused on obese adults) can be set aside in favour of the more applicable studies, i.e. those that are generalisable to the 10-year-old child.

We have looked at one question in detail, but the nurse may have a number of information needs relating to this patient. Some of the questions arising from these information needs are highlighted in Table 2.1.

TABLE 2.1 OTHER QUESTIONS ABOUT PREVENTION OR TREATMENT OF PRESSURE SORES

Population or problem	Intervention (or test or exposure)	Comparison intervention (if any)	Outcome
Patients with pressure sores (partial- or full-thickness skin loss)	Application of hydrocolloids	Application of gauze dressings	Reduced time to healing Faster shrinkage of the pressure sore
Patients with pressure sores (partial- or full-thickness skin loss)	Ascorbic acid supplementation	Usual diet with no additional supplements	Reduced time to healing Faster shrinkage of the pressure sore
Critically ill children	Constant low-pressure devices or alternating pressure devices	Three-hourly lifting or turning	Prevention of pressure sores, defined here as discolouration of the skin, or partial- or full-thickness skin loss Risk of destabilising the patient, poor cardiac output Costs

SCENARIO 2.2

Alison, a 2-year-old infant, presented at the local accident and emergency department with fever and vomiting. In line with departmental policy, urine was collected in a bag (which had been applied to her perineum according to the manufacturer's instructions), then sent for microscopy and culture. The white cell count was found to be high and Alison was started on a course of antibiotics. She was asked to return in 5 days, by which time the urine culture results would be available. At her follow-up appointment, the attending physician was frustrated to note that the culture results showed a mixed growth. It was not clear whether Alison had indeed suffered a urinary tract infection (UTI) or whether the urine sample had simply been contaminated. In view of the risk of underlying urinary tract abnormalities and potential upper urinary tract damage, children with UTI are investigated carefully. Concerned that the methods used for obtaining urine samples were inappropriate, the physician suggested that, in future, bag-catch urine sampling should be abandoned in favour of clean-catch urine sampling. This method requires that the infant's nappy is removed and their carer provided with a sterile container and instructed to watch for the opportunity to catch the urine. The nurses on the unit were worried about the implications of changing practice. They felt that carers might not be successful in capturing urine specimens, and that this would cause delays for patients and their families.

The nurses want to know:
  What is the best way of obtaining a urine specimen for culture, from a child?

We can check how focused the question is, by examining each component individually.

Population

The population of interest comprises children suspected of having UTI; however, the nurses may want to consider further refining the population. The results of a study carried out on older children (who may be able to obtain the urine specimen themselves) are likely to be different from those of a study carried out in children still wearing nappies.

Intervention (or test or exposure)

In this case, there are two interventions of interest: the method of urine sampling which is currently used (i.e. urine bag sampling) and the proposed method of 'clean-catch' sampling. It may be useful to include brief details of the exact methods used when obtaining bag-catch and clean-catch urine specimens, as these may differ from those used by researchers and this could affect the applicability of study results.

Comparison intervention

Next we will look at the comparison intervention. Comparing two or more methods is a useful way of reaching a decision about a practice change. When investigating the accuracy of a (new) diagnostic test, the new test is compared against a reference standard test to see how well the two tests agree. A reference standard test is considered to be 'the best available method for establishing the presence or absence of the condition of interest' and can be a single method or a combination of methods (Bossuyt et al 2003). Alternatives to reference standard tests are often sought where the reference standard tests are difficult to perform, invasive, costly, inconvenient or unacceptable to the patient.

The reference standard method for obtaining urine from infants and babies is suprapubic aspiration of urine directly from the bladder (Downs 1999). The procedure is invasive, uncomfortable for the infant, and can be tricky where infants are uncooperative.

Outcome

The key outcome of interest is contamination of the culture specimen. Other outcomes that the nurses may wish to consider are time taken to obtain specimen, acceptability to patient and family, and ease of use.

In summary:

- *Population*: Children suspected of having UTI, who are not yet toilet trained
- *Interventions*: Bag-catch urine specimens and clean-catch urine specimens
- *Comparison*: Suprapubic aspiration
- *Outcome*: Contaminated culture specimen, as indicated by bacterial growth in either the bag-catch or clean-catch specimens, not found in the suprapubic aspiration.

TABLE 2.2 OTHER QUESTIONS ABOUT DIAGNOSIS OF URINARY TRACT INFECTION

Population or problem	Intervention (or test or exposure)	Comparison intervention (if any)	Outcome
Children suspected of having UTI, who are not yet toilet trained	Clean-catch urine sampling using a sterile container	Suprapubic aspiration directly from bladder	Culture contamination
Obtaining urine samples from children who are not yet toilet trained	Clean-catch method	Bag-catch method	Time taken to successfully obtain urine sample, cost, parent satisfaction, nurse satisfaction

The revised question is:

In children suspected of having UTI, who are not yet toilet trained, what is the risk of culture contamination when urine is obtained by (i) bag-catch or (ii) clean-catch, as compared with urine obtained by suprapubic aspiration directly from the bladder?

The optimal *study design* for this question would be studies assessing diagnostic test accuracy (discussed in Chapter 5). Examples of additional questions relating to this scenario are given in Table 2.2.

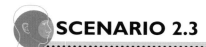 # SCENARIO 2.3

A recent public health report shows that despite national initiatives to promote breastfeeding, uptake is poor. A health visitor who works in a deprived, inner-city community and visits mothers from day 10 after delivery has noticed that many of the mothers feed their babies with infant milk formula rather than breast milk. The health visitor wants to gain a better under-standing of the factors that influence mothers to bottle feed with infant milk formula. This information may help to inform future educational programmes aimed at promoting breastfeeding.

The health visitor asks:
  Why do mothers not breastfeed?

The question does not easily fit the PICO formula, but it is nevertheless useful to consider each component of the question. It may be possible to further refine the question, thereby improving the chance of finding relevant research evidence.

Population

The health visitor works with mothers who live in a deprived area of the city, a population that has different needs and dif-ferent experiences to those of women in more affluent areas. In this case, the health visitor is interested in the views of moth-ers of all ages. If the problem were specific to very young, first-time mothers, the question would need to reflect this. The health visitor may find it useful to examine the views of both breast-feeding and bottle-feeding mothers in order to obtain informa-tion about the factors that influence mothers in their decision to breast- or bottle feed.

Intervention (or test or exposure)

Unlike questions relating to test accuracy or effectiveness of a treatment, there is no intervention for this type of question.

Outcomes

The health visitor is interested in mothers' perceptions, atti-tudes, values or beliefs relating to breastfeeding and/or to bottle feeding with infant formula.

The revised question is as follows:
  What are the factors, identified by mothers who live in deprived inner city areas, that influence them to breastfeed or to bottle feed using infant milk formula?

The *type of research* that is most likely to provide an in-depth understanding of the views of the mothers is qualitative research (discussed in Chapter 4).

Specific prompts for accessing research evidence

Healthcare practitioners should constantly evaluate their practice. New technologies (for example drugs, blood pressure monitoring devices, wound dressings) are introduced on a regular basis, different processes of care (case management, patient-held records, home care of long-term ventilated patients, etc.) are explored and new information (for example, factors associated with sudden infant death syndrome, literacy figures for the adult population, etc.) is published at regular intervals. A questioning approach to health care is important if such 'innovations' are to be identified in the first place and, secondly, if they are to be considered for inclusion in the management of patients. An attitude of 'research mindedness' (Perkins et al 1999, p. 4) is needed, asking questions such as 'Which is best?', 'Who should do this?', 'Where should this patient be treated?'. Blind acceptance of a technology that is skilfully marketed by a company representative, or outright rejection of change to an existing practice, could potentially impact negatively on patient outcome, resources and cost.

Although nurses would agree with the above, the need to access research evidence in the context of the clinical setting is not always apparent. One of the challenges for nurses and other healthcare professionals is to recognise the importance of asking questions about their practice.

Prompts for consulting scientific evidence include:

- uncertainty as to the best course of action
- controversy regarding the way a procedure or therapy should be carried out
- lack of knowledge about the effectiveness of one therapy or test over another
- unexpected patient outcomes

- the introduction of new therapies or technologies
- practices based on tradition
- 'novel' suggestions by patients.

For those aspects of care that are already entrenched in day-to-day practice, a questioning approach is equally important, but perhaps more difficult to achieve. Where a method of care delivery (for example, the 'drugs round' where drugs are dispensed to all ward patients at set times by a designated nurse) has become entrenched as routine practice, practitioners may accept it as the right or only method, and alternatives may not be considered. In addition, 'ritualistic' practices must be examined for clinical and cost effectiveness.

It may be helpful for the nurse to consider whether 'the right person is doing the right thing, in the right way, in the right place, at the right time, with the right result' (Graham 1996). By asking this question, any information gaps will be highlighted. Finally, reflection, a strategy used within nursing to encourage learning from practical experiences (Boud et al 1985), can be used as another method for identifying information needs. By their reflecting on 'critical incidents', any gaps in a nurse's knowledge of current research findings can be identified.

Prioritising questions

The volume of decisions and related need for information that arise each day can be overwhelming. It may be necessary to prioritise the questions for which best evidence is to be sought. Questions that are most important to the patient's well-being, that arise repeatedly (Sackett et al 1997) or that have potentially important consequences (such as risk or cost reductions) could be considered high-priority questions. At the Evidence-Based Child Health Unit in Liverpool, topics are prioritised according to:

- their relevance to the hospital and to NHS priorities
- whether they affect a significant number of patients

- potential to implement change in practice
- demand for the topic from a number of independent sources
- wide variations in practice
- genuine uncertainty or controversy as to best practice.

Questions for research

In the spirit of evidence-based practice, this chapter has focused on questions that nurses in the clinical field are asking; questions which they hope can be answered to some extent by previously published research evidence. However, the same PICO formula can be applied to many research questions (that may or may not arise directly from an interaction with a patient or clinical problem). In research, as with evidence-based practice, the question drives the research project. Asking a general, unfocused question will lead to difficulties at each step of the research process.

Questions and research evidence aren't enough

Our day-to-day clinical decisions are influenced (consciously or unconsciously) by a number of factors (Box 2.4). Although each of these factors is influential in its own right, when used in isolation, they may result in inappropriate decisions. The application of scientific evidence without considered judgement results in a 'cookbook' approach to health care, with nurses following 'recipes' for care regardless of the patient's specific needs. In contrast, over-reliance on personal experience when making decisions can be equally damaging. For example, if practice nurses continue to recommend bed rest to people with acute lower back pain because it appears to have worked in the past, they will be ignoring evidence that bed rest is less effective in reducing pain and improving an individual's ability to perform everyday activities than advice to stay active (Hagen et al 2004). In people with type 2 diabetes mellitus, one-off routine annual testing of urine may be the usual practice; however, evidence indicates that a single

---

BOX 2.4 Factors influencing the decision-making process

Up-to-date research evidence
Clinical expertise:
— formal education
— accumulated knowledge (journal articles, textbooks, press reports, expert opinion, advice from colleagues, clinical audit)
— past experience built on a case-by-case basis
— pattern recognition, intuition
— most recent experience
— skill level
Beliefs, attitudes, values, tradition
Routine, 'the way things are done around here'
Factors relating to the patient and their family:
— clinical circumstances, co-morbid conditions
— preferences, values, beliefs, attitudes, expectations, concerns
— needs
Organisational factors
— national and local policies
— service/resource availability
— funding
— equipment
— time

---

annual near-patient test is not sufficiently sensitive in identifying people with renal disease. Instead urine should be tested at least annually and on more than one occasion for proteinuria and, if found to be negative, it should subsequently be tested for microalbuminuria (NHS CRD 2000).

Up-to-date, valid evidence, directly relevant to the situation at hand, needs to be integrated together with the other influencing factors in order to maximise the likelihood of the expected outcome being achieved.

Exercise

We encourage you to consolidate your learning by undertaking the worked exercise on the website.

Summary

The success or failure of explicitly basing nursing practice on best evidence relies on nurses challenging both new and established methods of caring for patients. The skills provided in this chapter, summarised in Box 2.5, provide a starting point for seeking out good-quality evidence to support current practice or a change in practice. Numerous opportunities for practising these skills will present themselves during the course of the working day. This first step in the evidence-based process is an important one, and nurses who take the time to develop carefully worded questions will be well rewarded at each stage in the process.

BOX 2.5 Quick reference: applying your new skills in clinical practice

- Consider what additional information is required when making a health care decision.
- Prioritise which information you need to address.
- Formulate a question.
- Focus the question using the PICO formula.
- Decide how specific or how general each part of the question needs to be.
- Decide which study design is most likely to provide valid results.
- Refer to the focused question at each stage of the evidence-based process, i.e. when searching for or appraising evidence, and when applying the evidence to your situation.

References

Bandolier Glossary, 2004. Selection bias. Available online at: www.jr2.ox.ac.uk/bandolier/glossary.html. November 2010.

Bossuyt, P.M., Reitsma, J.B., Bruns, D.E., et al., 2003. Towards complete and accurate reporting of studies of diagnostic accuracy: the STARD Initiative. Radiology 226, 24–28.

Boud, D., Keogh, R., Walker, D., 1985. Reflection: turning experience into learning. Kogan Page, London.

Bryman, A., 1988. Quantity and quality in social research. Unwin Hyman, London.

Burton, M.J., Doree, C.J., 2003. Ear drops for the removal of ear wax. Cochrane Database Syst. Rev. 2003 (3). Art. No.: CD004326. doi:10.1002/14651858.CD004326.

Bury, T.J., Mead, J.M. (Eds.), 1998. Evidence based healthcare: a practical guide for therapists. Butterworth-Heinemann, Oxford.

Clegg, A.J., Loveman, E., Gospodarevskaya, E., et al., 2010. The safety and effectiveness of different methods of earwax removal: a systematic review and economic evaluation. Health Technol. Assess. 14 (28), 1–192.

Cullum, N., Deeks, J., Sheldon, T.A., Song, F., Fletcher, A.W., 2000. Beds, mattresses and cushions for pressure sore prevention and treatment (Cochrane Review). Cochrane Library 2000 (3). Update Software, Oxford 3.

Dinsdale, R.C., Roland, P.S., Manning, S.C., 1991. Catastrophic otologic injury from oral jet irrigation of the external auditory canal. Laryngoscope 101, 75–78.

Downs, S.M., 1999. Technical report: urinary tract infections in febrile infants and young children. Pediatrics 103 (4), e54.

Graham, G., 1996. Clinically effective medicine in a rational health service. Health Director (June), 11–12.

Greenhalgh, T., 1997. How to read a paper – the basics of evidence based medicine. BMJ Publishing, London.

Hagen, K., Hilde, G., Jamtvedt, G., Winnem, M., 2004. Bedrest for acute low back pain and sciatica. Cochrane Database Syst. Rev. 2004 (4). Art. No.: CD001254. doi:10.1002/14651858. CD001254. pub2.

Laupacis, A., Wells, G., Scott Richardson, W., Tugwell, P., for the Evidence-Based Medicine Working Group, 1994. Users' guides to the medical literature. How to use an article about prognosis. JAMA 272 (3), 234–237. Available online at: www.cche.net/ usersguides/prognosis.asp. November 2010.

Logan, S., Gilbert, R., 2000. Framing questions. In: Moyer, V.A., Elliot, E.J., Davis, R.L., et al. (Eds.), Evidence based paediatrics and child health. BMJ Books, London.

NHS CRD (Centre for Reviews and Dissemination), 2000. Complications of diabetes: renal disease and promotion of self-management. Effective Health Care Bulletin 6 (1), 1–12.

Perkins, E.R., Simnett, I., Wright, L., 1999. Creative tensions in evidence-based practice. In: Perkins, E.R., Simnett, I., Wright, L. (Eds.), Evidence based health promotion. Wiley, New York.

Price, J., 1997. Problems of ear syringing. Practice Nurse 14 (2), 126–127.

Sackett, D.L., Richardson, W.S., Rosenberg, W., Haynes, R.B., 1997. Evidence based medicine: how to practice and teach EBM. Churchill Livingstone, New York.

Sackett, D.L., Strauss, S.E., Richardson, W.S., Rosenberg, W., Haynes, R.B., 2000. Evidence-based medicine: how to practise and teach EBM, second ed. Churchill Livingstone, London.

Sharp, J.F., Wilson, J.A., Ross, L., Barr-Hamilton, R.M., 1990. Ear wax removal: a survey of current practice. Br. Med. J. 301, 1251–1252.

Zikk, D., Rappaport, Y., Himelfarb, M.Z., 1991. Invasive external otitis after removal of impacted cerumen by irrigation. N. Engl. J. Med. 325, 969–970.

Zivic, R.C., King, S., 1993. Cerumen-impaction management for clients of all ages. Nurse Pract. 18 (3), 29–39.

CHAPTER 3

Searching the literature

Olwen Beaven and Jean V Craig

KEY POINTS

- Identifying best evidence requires an understanding of basic search principles. More advanced techniques will help to enhance a search.

- To identify research evidence in the most efficient way, start with a focused question, select databases that are most likely to yield information about your question, and build a search strategy using appropriate search terms, combined in the right way.

- Databases/resources are best searched in order of usefulness.

- Techniques to limit the number of irrelevant articles retrieved (such as searching using index terms only, where available) are invaluable.

- Systematic reviews require extensive searching and it is advisable to obtain specialist advice on building comprehensive search strategies for each of the resources to be searched.

- The internet can be a valuable source of information, especially if reliable/ quality-assessed resources are used.

Introduction

The purpose of this chapter is to provide a beginner's guide to the principles and practice of searching the research literature. Whilst it is unrealistic to teach the art of searching within the constraints of the printed page, it is possible to pass on a basic understanding of the search process and the core competencies needed to enable readers to develop the skills required for efficiently identifying research evidence. The importance of searching the literature to find information is often overlooked in the hurry to find an answer; however, a good literature search can underpin the whole problem-solving process. If key information is missing it is much harder to identify an appropriate solution to a clinical question.

Although this chapter is primarily aimed at novice searchers, it provides useful revision for the more confident searcher and includes sections specifically for the advanced searcher.

We start the chapter with an overview of basic search principles applied to database searching and then discuss a systematic approach for retrieving the most useful evidence, targeting, for example, resources that contain 'pre-appraised' evidence in the first instance. We present useful sources of evidence, and show an example search on one of these sources (the MEDLINE database). We then give additional tips and techniques for refining a search, and flag up the complexities of undertaking the comprehensive searching required for systematic review purposes.

Where is research information found?

The large number of journals produced around the world precludes searching for individual articles by hand. Journal indexes have, therefore, been converted onto electronic databases. These bibliographic databases gather together articles within a particular subject category such as engineering, sociology, history, medicine or agriculture. The CINAHL database, for example, provides a cumulative index of nursing and allied health literature.

Databases are produced in a variety of formats: CDROM versions, worldwide web/internet options and, in many organisations, databases are 'networked' onto all the computers. Regardless of format, organisations have to pay to access databases so a limited range only may be made available in any one organisation.

Most databases provide similar information about each included article (or 'record'); usually the title, author, where it was published (the journal, year, volume, issue and page numbers) and the short abstract/summary, if available. Databases do not normally contain the full text of the whole article, although, increasingly, free full-text articles are becoming available electronically.

Each section of a journal article (title, author, abstract, etc.) in a database is called a 'field'. Each new field starts with a two-letter code to make it clearly identifiable. For example, a typical record in a bibliographic database might look something like this:

TI: The joys of nursing
AU: Anybody G. C., Somebody H. L., Other A. N.
SO: Supernurse, 1997, 15 (2); 378–84
PY: 1997
AB: There have been numerous campaigns over recent years to boost the recruitment of young people into the nursing profession. These have taken a variety of approaches and have focused on different aspects of the job, from how challenging nursing is, to the rewards of watching a patient recover from illness/injury. This paper looks at the positive images of nursing portrayed in these advertising campaigns and compares them with the reality as perceived by nurses currently employed.
UI: SN9725938

Getting help with database searching

Hospital libraries are an obvious port of call for obtaining training, advice or self-help tutorials on literature searching. Librarians will often help you to focus your question, to construct the search and to select which databases to search. Increasingly, librarians are offering an information service whereby they conduct the search for articles relevant to a particular clinical question. Such services are extremely useful but acquiring the skills to conduct your own searches will prove invaluable in terms of day-to-day clinical decision-making.

Basic search principles

Although databases are produced by different companies and so vary in terms of subject matter and layout, they all tend to require the same general approach to searching. The key principle in searching is to match words that describe your question or topic of interest with journal articles containing the same (or very similar) words, in the hope that these journal articles address your topic/question of interest. This section looks at some basic theory that can be applied to searching most databases.

Analysing the question

When starting a literature search, it is important to have a clear question in mind so the exact information required can be identified in the most efficient way. The first step in developing a search strategy is to break a question down into its key components (see the PICO question formulation process described in Chapter 2). Think about the Population, the Interventions/therapies/tests/exposures, any Comparison interventions and specific Outcomes covered by a question. An example is given in Box 3.1.

BOX 3.1 Key components of a question

Question: In people with needle phobia, what are the effects of non-pharmacological interventions on their fear or anxiety associated with needles and injections?

Population:	People with fear of needles
Intervention(s):	Differing types of behavioural therapy
Comparison:	One behavioural therapy intervention compared with another
Outcome:	Fear/anxiety

Search terms

Having established the key PICO components of a question, generate a word list for each component.

Free text

In free text searching, you build word lists of all the different terms that an author may use to describe a key component of the search, including plural and singular words, synonyms, abbreviations, variations in spellings, possible hyphenation and any regularly used non-English language terms. Be cautious when using abbreviations. A search for articles using the abbreviation 'AIDS', for example, will identify articles looking at hearing aids, mobility aids, etc., as well as articles on autoimmune deficiency syndrome. If too many irrelevant articles are retrieved from a search incorporating abbreviations, you may want to consider re-running the search without these abbreviated terms.

The lists for each component may be fairly comprehensive as shown in Box 3.2.

BOX 3.2 Suggested word lists for the question on needle phobia

Population:	Fear, phobia
	Needles, syringes, injection(s), hypodermic(s)
Interventions:	Behavio(u)r(al) therapy, relaxation, coping
	skills, cognitive therapy, hypnotherapy, hypnosis,
	psychotherapy, distraction, diversion (and so on)
Comparison:	(Same as interventions)
Outcomes:	Alleviation or reduction of fear/stress/anxiety, stress
	relief, calm, relaxed

Type the list of words for one or more of the PICO components into the search window, combining the words with the appropriate linking word (as explained below). The database then matches this combination of words to records containing the same words anywhere within the abstract, title or author fields (or, in some databases, anywhere within the record).

A search using free text usually has a high recall rate or high sensitivity (i.e. large numbers of records are retrieved by the search), but a low precision rate or low specificity (i.e. many of the retrieved records are irrelevant) (NHS CRD 2001). This is because in free text searching, any record containing the free text words is retrieved, even if the words are used to discuss a very minor detail within the record. To increase precision of the search, albeit at the expense of sensitivity, a search using index terms only (see below) can be carried out.

Index terms

These are keywords that are added onto each journal article by the database producers to reflect the most important topics covered by that record. To illustrate, articles within a specific database that contain the terms breast cancer, breast carcinoma or breast tumour would all be assigned the unique index term: 'breast neoplasm'. It does not matter which words the authors of an article use to describe the topic; if the research publication focuses on breast cancer, it will always be labelled with the index term 'breast neoplasm', within that database.

When searching for articles on this topic, instead of having to think of all the different terms that authors might use, as is the case with free text searching, the appropriate index term can be used instead. A further important benefit of index terms is that journal articles that briefly mention a topic will not be retrieved when index terms only are used. This is because index terms are assigned only to those topics which form a large part of the record. A search using index terms – also known as controlled vocabulary searching – is, therefore, more precise (has a higher specificity) than a search using free text terms. A disadvantage of using index terms only is that any records that have not been appropriately indexed may be missed by the search.

To find the index term, you usually access the thesaurus provided in the database. Information on use of the thesaurus is given on page 77, under Step 2 of the example search of Medline database (PubMed version).

Combined free text and controlled vocabulary (index) searching

Some databases automatically match free text search terms to appropriate index terms, thereby retrieving records through a combination of free text and controlled vocabulary searching. The help section of the database will clarify whether or not this is done.

Linking word lists (Boolean logic: AND, OR, NOT)

Search terms are linked together to get the combination of components needed for a question using the terms AND and OR.

AND combines words together, so that both words must appear within one article to be found by a search (Fig. 3.1). A search for 'needles AND fear' will find only those articles that contain both the words needles and fear.

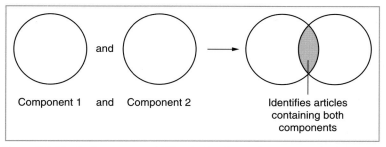

Figure 3.1 The Boolean operator AND only identifies articles containing both specified components

OR enables selection of any one of a number of specified words/ phrases in a list, so that if either one or another specified word/ phrase appears in an article, it will be found in a search (Fig. 3.2). A search for 'behavioural OR behavioral OR behaviour OR behavior OR relaxation OR hypnotherapy OR hypnosis OR distraction' will find articles containing at least one of the words/ phrases in the list.

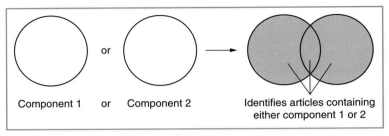

Figure 3.2 The Boolean operator OR identifies articles containing either specified component

It is also possible to exclude specific words/phrases from a search so articles containing them will not be identified. This is done using the term NOT (Fig. 3.3). A search for 'fear of needles NOT fear of hospitals' will find articles containing the phrase 'fear of needles' that do not also contain the phrase 'fear of hospitals'. Be very cautious when using NOT, as it can inadvertently exclude articles that are relevant to a question.

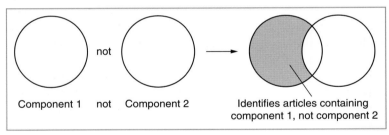

Figure 3.3 The Boolean operator NOT identifies articles containing one specified component but not the other specified component

AND, OR and NOT, in this context, are known as 'Boolean logic operators'.

Additional search techniques commonly available

Applying some additional search techniques can help to further refine the search strategy.

Phrase searching

If, for example, you are looking for articles on *pressure sores*, you will want to avoid retrieving those articles that discuss *pressure* and *sores* separately, as such articles are unlikely to address your information need. In some databases, a search for *pressure sore* will retrieve records where the words *pressure* and *sore* appear anywhere in the record, but not necessarily next to each other, thereby increasing the number of irrelevant records retrieved. For these databases, it is necessary to enclose the phrase in quotes (*"pressure sore"*) or to use some other technique to force retrieval of articles that use the exact phrase *pressure sore*. The help option within the database will explain which technique to use.

Truncation

Many databases will retrieve only those records that contain the *exact* word or phrase that you have typed. Truncation is a short-cut device that avoids you having to type out all the different variations of a word when free text searching. You type the stem of a word followed by the truncation symbol, often denoted by a * or $ in databases. The 'help' option within the database will explain which symbol should be used for truncation. A draw-back is that truncation reduces the precision of the search:

- ulcer$ would pick up ulcer, ulcers, ulceration, ulcerated, etc. (all potentially relevant to sickle cell leg ulcers), but also ulcer-carcinoma, ulcero-bubonic and many other words that have nothing to do with that topic.
- 'Bab*' would pick up baby and babies, but also other words like baboon, babesiosis, babble, babesia, Babinski reflex, etc.

Wildcard

The 'wildcard', available on some databases, allows you to search for words with alternative spellings without having to type out each word in full. The wildcard is inserted in the word where extra or alternative letter(s) might be placed. It is often denoted by a ? in databases:

- an?emia would pick up both anaemia and anemia
- wom?n would pick up both woman and women.

Where to search first

Having clarified a question and identified the words necessary to search for relevant information, the next step is to identify the resources most likely to contain articles relevant to that question, and to consider the order in which they should be searched.

Since the advent and expansion of the internet, it is tempting to dive online and see what can be found via a preferred internet browser. Whilst this simplicity is attractive, it is not the best way to identify well-conducted research evidence appropriate for use in clinical settings. The internet is an open and unregulated resource. There is no quality control of websites so the information provided can be biased, unfounded and misleading, just as easily as it can be accurate and well-balanced. Rather than exploring such a vast pool of information of unknown quality and validity, it is considered more productive to have a structured and organised approach that focuses on more reliable and established resources first.

Haynes (2001) put forward the idea of hierarchy of sources of evidence (further refined by DiCenso et al in 2009), suggesting that the most effective way to search the research literature is to focus on healthcare resources at the top of the '6S' hierarchy and then work methodically down through each level until the information required is found (Fig. 3.4).

Systems

At the top of the '6S' hierarchy are technical/automated systems – not yet in widespread use – that, for example, link into a patient's electronic record and offer up-to-date, computerised decision support for their particular clinical condition.

Summaries

Evidence-based guidelines and other resources that integrate, evaluate and concisely summarise important research evidence about a clinical problem form the next level in the hierarchy.

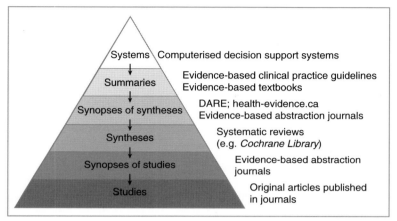

Figure 3.4 The 6S hierarchy of pre-appraised evidence (DiCenso et al. 2009). (From DiCenso A, Bayley L, Haynes B. Accessing pre-appraised evidence: fine-tuning the 5S model into a 6S model. In *Evidence Based Nursing* (2009) 12;4:99–101, with permission from BMJ Publishing Group Ltd.)

Examples of organisations producing guidelines with explicit, rigorous methods include the Scottish Intercollegiate Guidelines Network (SIGN: www.sign.ac.uk) and the National Institute for Health and Clinical Excellence (NICE: www.nice.org.uk). Guidelines are generated by many different healthcare organisations and professional bodies, so websites such as the National Guideline Clearinghouse (from the US Agency for Health care Research and Quality: www.guideline.gov), or NHS Evidence (where retrieved articles can be filtered by 'types of information' to yield guidelines only: http://www.evidence.nhs.uk/default.aspx), are useful first ports of call for tracking down good-quality guidelines. Guideline resources may have a specialised focus (for example, NHS Clinical Knowledge Summaries – http://www.cks.nhs.uk/home – are aimed at primary healthcare professionals), whilst others are more generic (see, for example, *Health Evidence Bulletins Wales* at http://hebw.cf.ac.uk/).

Commercial evidence summary products include *Clinical Evidence* from the BMJ (http://clinicalevidence.bmj.com/ceweb/index.jsp), *UpToDate* (http://www.uptodate.com/home/index.html) and *DynaMed* (http://www.ebscohost.com/dynamed/). The range of medical conditions covered by these products and the methods of evaluation used when compiling these resources vary. Libraries will be able to advise if access to these resources has been purchased.

The Joanna Briggs Institute originating in Australia presents summaries of best practice for a variety of clinical topics relevant to nursing. Its *Best Practice Information Sheets* can be accessed at http://www.joannabriggs.edu.au/pubs/best_practice.php

Synopses of syntheses

If consultation with resources at the top of the 6S hierarchy does not yield a solution, the next level to check includes the synopses of systematic reviews. Systematic reviews use systematic and explicit methods to identify, select, critically appraise and synthesise the available research evidence pertinent to a specified question (see Chapter 7 for more information). Synopses of systematic reviews report only essential information, in a format that allows the reader to quickly ascertain the quality of the study (the synopsis includes a quality appraisal) and its key messages.

The journal *Evidence-Based Nursing* (http://ebn.bmj.com/) provides research abstracts and expert commentary on the clinical application of systematic reviews (and other research studies) that have met certain quality criteria, and that are applicable to nursing practice. Other journals in this genre include *Evidence-Based Medicine*, *Evidence-Based Mental Health* and *Evidence-Based Dentistry*. The Knowledge Library within *Bandolier* (http://www.medicine.ox.ac.uk/bandolier/knowledge.html) is a collection of abstracted information from good-quality systematic reviews or individual studies, grouped according to clinical topic. Each report contains additional information, compiled by the team at *Bandolier*, about the importance of the study and/or what it means in terms of clinical practice.

Syntheses

If neither summaries of collected evidence nor synopses of systematic reviews are available, the next level in the hierarchy comprises full-text individual systematic reviews. If a systematic review addresses your question, then the effort of searching for individual studies, ascertaining the quality and findings of those studies, and pulling together (often contradictory) results from the individual studies, is saved. In the absence of a trustworthy synopsis of the systematic review, you will still need to appraise the review for methodological quality, clinical importance and applicability, but this is easier than appraising and assimilating the data from numerous studies.

The Cochrane Library

The first place to check for systematic reviews in health care is *The Cochrane Library*, a collection of six databases that contain different types of high-quality, independent evidence to inform healthcare decision-making. The search interface allows for all of these databases to be searched simultaneously from the opening screen (Fig. 3.5). The most useful databases for identifying systematic reviews are the Cochrane Database of Systematic Reviews (labelled "Cochrane Reviews") and the Database of Abstracts of Reviews of Effects (DARE) (labelled "Other Reviews"). The Cochrane Database of Systematic Reviews contains the full text of systematic reviews conducted by the Cochrane Collaboration. These are primarily systematic reviews of studies investigating the effectiveness of healthcare interventions, but systematic reviews of diagnostic test accuracy studies are now also becoming available.

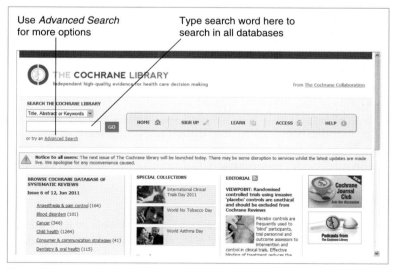

Figure 3.5 The Cochrane Library opening screen. (Reproduced by kind permission of Wiley-Blackwell Ltd.)

Cochrane systematic reviews are updated at intervals to incorporate latest research evidence and are subject to rigorous peer review. DARE ("Other Reviews") is produced by the Centre for Reviews and Dissemination (CRD) in York, UK. It contains structured abstracts and critical appraisals of non-Cochrane systematic reviews but not the full text of these reviews.

The Cochrane Library is published online and in DVD format. A detailed user guide and other teaching materials for the internet version are available from the website ("http://www.thecochrane library.com/view/0/HowtoUse.html"). DARE is also freely available at the CRD website - "http://www.crd.york.ac.uk/crdweb/" (select the DARE tab: Database of Abstracts of Reviews of Effects).

The Campbell Collaboration

For evidence-based questions that cross into more social- or behavioural-oriented interventions, there are the resources of the Campbell Collaboration. This is a 'sister' organisation to the Cochrane Collaboration. The Campbell Library holds the Campbell Collaboration's collection of systematic reviews in education, crime and justice, and social welfare and is available via the Campbell Collaboration website (http://www.campbell-collaboration.org/library.php).

Synopses of studies and studies

If, at this stage, no good-quality publications have been found, then synopses of individual studies or, failing that, full-text individual studies are looked for. Individual studies are at the bottom of the hierarchy, because they don't have the 'added value' of the integrated, summarised and pre-appraised resources.

Useful databases

Staff at hospital/university libraries should be able to give advice about any bibliographic databases they subscribe to. Standard bibliographic databases for individual research studies in the health care/nursing field include, for example:

- MEDLINE (a general medical database, produced in the USA). There are a number of versions available. PubMed is the free internet version which comes direct from the creators of MEDLINE (the National Library of Medicine in the USA). Later on in this chapter we show an example search on PubMed
- CINAHL (Cumulative Index of Nursing and Allied Health Literature, a general nursing database, produced in the USA)
- EMBASE (a general medical database, produced in Europe; more foreign language material)
- Within the Cochrane Library (see above), the *Clinical Trials* database (also known as *Cochrane Central Register of Controlled Trials (CENTRAL)*). This is the most comprehensive bibliographic database of randomised controlled trials (RCTs) and possible RCTs in health care. If no systematic reviews are found to answer the question of interest, and if the optimum study design for the question is the RCT (as in questions about effectiveness of an intervention or investigation), then this is an excellent source of evidence
- The Campbell Collaboration (see above) holds a register of RCTs (and possible RCTs) in education, social work and welfare, and criminal justice (C2-SPECTR)
- Many topic-specific databases are available, such as PsycINFO, AgeLine, PEDro (physiotherapy evidence database). A comprehensive list of databases is provided in Section 6.2 of the Cochrane Handbook for Systematic Reviews of Interventions, available at http://cochrane-handbook.org/ and Appendix 3.1 lists some examples of databases.

All these databases are produced by different companies/organisations so they will often look different, contain different information, and the specific searching tools available may vary. There will be variation between CD-ROM, internet and 'online' versions.

Which databases you choose to search will depend on factors such as:

- the specific subject of a search
- availability
- how easy/difficult it is to search.

It is helpful to find out as much as possible about any databases that are available (check search tools, etc.) and to do a quick test search to see how useful they are in practice.

Always make a note of which database(s) are searched, the years/date searched, the version(s), and the search terms used, for each question or project that is undertaken. This is particularly useful if, at any time in the future, the search is to be rerun. It also serves as a reminder of how extensive the search was.

Online search tools to assist finding evidence from this hierarchy

Although we have provided examples of sources of evidence for each level of the 6S hierarchy above, you may find it useful to search across a number of databases simultaneously, without having to log onto each database individually.

'Search engines' such as Google, Alta Vista, Yahoo and Lycos, and 'meta-search engines' such as SavvySearch and MetaCrawler are often used by healthcare professionals and patients to find information on specific diseases or interventions. However, these 'generic' type search engines produce lists of thousands of web pages that best match the search terms used and many of the retrieved web pages will not have a research focus. It is, therefore, preferable to use search engines that specifically target databases of recognised medical research publications. Google Scholar is one example; using the advanced search option, you can restrict your search to a particular subject area, for example, medicine, pharmacology and veterinary science or social sciences, arts and humanities. Arguably more useful than Google Scholar, are TRIP and SUMSearch, which group search results by category, as discussed below.

TRIP (Turning Research into Practice) database

TRIP searches a broad range of evidence-based healthcare-related websites including *Effective Healthcare Bulletins*, NHS CRD Reports, *Bandolier*, the Cochrane Library databases, the *Evidence-Based* Journals mentioned previously and many others. The search screen is very simple to use. Just type in the word or phrase to be identified and when the search has been completed, a list of Results by Category (evidence based, guidelines, medical images, etc.) is displayed. Choose a category and a list of relevant items is presented, with the name of the resource in which they were found. Click on items one by one to view them. The TRIP database can be searched at: www .tripdatabase.com/.

SUMSearch

This is a search system devised by the University of Texas, Health Science Center at San Antonio. When search term(s) are typed in, this system will automatically check (internet versions of) MEDLINE, DARE, the National Guideline Clearinghouse from the Agency for Health Care Policy and Research (AHCPR), an online textbook (usually the Merck Manual) and a few other databases depending on the topic. SUMSearch uses the MeSH (MEDLINE) thesaurus, so index terms as well as free text terms can be used to search. The search screen is straightforward to use and the system makes suggestions to help produce an accurate search. Search results are split into two types: broad/general discussions of the topic, or systematic reviews and original research. SUMSearch can be found at http://sumsearch.org/.

Other gateways to healthcare information

In England, NHS Evidence (www.evidence.nhs.uk) provides easy access to carefully selected evidence-based resources. A search of all resources can be conducted simultaneously from the home page, and the search results selected by, for example, types of information. An understanding of the 6S hierarchy of evidence comes to the fore here; to retrieve information near the top of the hierarchy, limit the search to guidelines or to systematic reviews by clicking on the appropriate filter on the left hand side of the search page. NHS Evidence also allows for more concentrated searching via the 'Conduct a specialist search' link.

Similarly, Health on the Net Northern Ireland (HONNI) (http://www.honni.qub.ac.uk/), The Knowledge Network NHS Scotland (http://www.knowledge.scot.nhs.uk/home.aspx), and Health in Wales Information Service (HOWIS) (http://www.wales.nhs.uk/) all typically provide access to evidence-based resources, guidelines, databases, electronic journals and books, etc. Some items are freely available but others will require passwords, which hospital libraries should be able to provide. These library-style collections of resources, made accessible through one website, are increasingly becoming the best places to start looking for information. Equivalent 'national electronic library sites' are probably available to those working in other countries too. Staff at local hospital libraries should be able to provide advice on such resources.

There are also some subject-specific 'gateway' sites, set up to serve groups of academics, researchers, students and others wanting information in that field. For example, Intute is run by a consortium of UK Universities and other partners and offers a free online service to help find the best web resources for research and study. A number of their gateways are relevant to the healthcare sector:

- Medicine including Dentistry: This gateway is designed to direct viewers to health and medicine web pages that have been assessed and met the desired quality standard. It also provides some self-help tutorials on searching the internet, as well as links to sites that match its quality criteria. It can be accessed at: www.intute.ac.uk/medicine/

- Nursing, Midwifery and Allied Health: This gateway focuses specifically on identifying quality websites related to nursing, midwifery and the allied health professions. It can be found at: www.intute.ac.uk/nmah/

- Psychology: This gateway provides links to quality assessed websites related to psychology including mental health. It can be found at: www.intute.ac.uk/psychology/

- Social Science: This gateway links to quality websites related to the social sciences. Of particular relevance to health care is the coverage of social welfare (including community care and carers) and education. It can be found at: www.intute.ac.uk/socialsciences

Lists and links to healthcare websites

Some groups provide lists of websites on certain subject areas to help people identify sites of possible interest. For evidence-based health care there is an excellent list provided by ScHARR (the School of Health and Related Research), at Sheffield University, known as 'Netting the Evidence – A ScHARR Introduction to Evidence Based Practice on the Internet'. It consists of a list of evidence-based healthcare websites, each with an accompanying description, providing useful background about each site. 'Netting the Evidence' can be found at www.shef.ac.uk/scharr/ir/netting/.

The other approach to finding sites of interest is to go to the websites of established organisations and look at their 'useful links' webpages. In evidence-based health care, organisations such as the NHS Centre for Reviews and Dissemination, the Cochrane Collaboration, the Centre for Evidence Based Nursing, etc., all have web pages. In the nursing field there are sites for the Royal College of Nursing, the Royal College of Midwives, etc.

See Appendix 3.2 for further information.

Further advice on internet resources and searching

Whilst printed resources on internet searching can become out of date quite quickly (especially given the ever-changing environment of the internet), they may provide helpful guidance on particular aspects of searching. Some examples of resources include:

- Pallen M 1998 Guide to the internet: an introduction for healthcare professionals, 2nd edn. BMJ Publishing, London
- Anon 1999 Health Net: a health and wellness guide to the internet, 2nd edn. McGraw-Hill, London
- Kiley R 2003 Medical information on the internet: a guide for health professionals, 3rd edn. Churchill Livingstone, Edinburgh
- Nicoll L H 2001 Computers in Nursing: Nurses' guide to the internet, 3rd edn. Lippincott, Philadelphia

Two examples of internet-based tutorials are:

- Bare Bones 101, from the University of South Carolina, Beaufort Library. This provides a basic tutorial on searching the internet. It can be found at: www.sc.edu/beaufort/library/pages/bones/bones.shtml.
- Internet for Nursing. This is a teach-yourself tutorial on internet research skills. It can be found at: www.vts.intute.ac.uk/tutorial/nursing.

Reflecting on resources

We hope the preceding section has prompted you to take a considered approach when selecting which resources to access. Box 3.3 highlights some of the key points that we have discussed.

BOX 3.3 Key points to remember about where to search first

1. Check with your hospital or university library to identify which resources you have access to and to obtain support and advice in using them.
2. When searching for research evidence, take account of the hierarchy of evidence.
3. Summaries of evidence (such as evidence-based guidelines) and synopses of systematic reviews bring together all the relevant evidence in a concise and convenient package for busy clinicians to use.
4. Resort to searching for individual research articles only if more useful, 'value-added' evidence (such as a well conducted evidence-based guidelines, synopsis of a systematic review or a systematic review) cannot be identified.
5. Use established bibliographic databases (organisations may have to pay for access) or use their equivalent internet versions.
6. Use health-related 'gateway' sites or subject lists/links compiled by reliable groups/organisations, in preference to generic search engines, to find healthcare research.

An example search on the MEDLINE database (PubMed version)

This next section looks at the process of undertaking a search on the MEDLINE database. MEDLINE is available in a variety of versions including PubMed, OVID, Dialogue and Silver Platter. We have used the PubMed version in our example. PubMed is developed by the National Center for Biotechnology Information at the US National Library of Medicine, and can be accessed free of charge at www.ncbi.nlm.nih.gov/sites/entrez?db=pubmed. PubMed provides numerous methods of searching, only some of which are described below. For further information on using this database, click on the the PubMed FAQs (frequently asked questions)/PubMed Tutorials links located on the home page screen (Fig. 3.6). The tutorial offers an interactive training programme. Most healthcare databases provide detailed information on search techniques, so you should find it easy to adapt the process described below to any database.

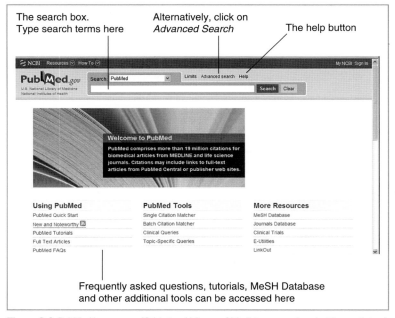

Figure 3.6 PubMed home page (© National Library of Medicine, reproduced with permission.)

Search terms can be entered into the Search Box of the home page (a screen shot is shown in Fig. 3.6.) or the Advanced Search page accessed via the Advanced search link. We prefer to work from the Advanced Search page (Fig. 3.7) as it offers more options. We use the question on needle phobia from the Basic search principles section (Box 3.1) to build a search specifically designed for PubMed. Some controlled vocabulary searching, i.e. use of index terms, as well as free text searching is used.

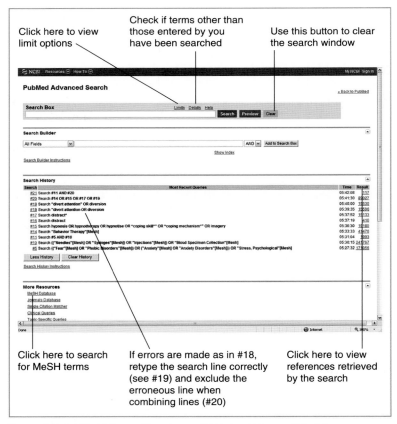

Figure 3.7 PubMed Advanced Search page (© National Library of Medicine, reproduced with permission.)

Step 1: checking what search tools are available

First check the search tools available in the database. This will usually be under the help information in the database (look for a 'help' button or heading). Check which words the database uses for Boolean logic. They are often AND, OR and NOT, but not always. Check also whether they are case sensitive (i.e. whether or not you need to use capital letters). Check for the symbols used for truncation and the wildcard if available and check whether a phrase has to be specified in any way, for example by using quotation marks.

In PubMed, the Boolean operators are AND, OR and NOT (upper case); the truncation symbol is *; phrases should be enclosed in double quotes.

Step 2: using the thesaurus

Use the thesaurus to see whether there are any indexing terms that correspond to the concepts identified in your question.

The thesaurus in PubMed is known as the MeSH® (Medical Subject Headings) thesaurus. MeSH® is a registered trademark of the United States National Library of Medicine. In PubMed, free text terms are automatically matched to appropriate MeSH (index) terms (where available), provided truncation is not used. So, a search using free text terms will automatically retrieve records containing the exact typed words/phrases as well as records that have been assigned the relevant MeSH (index) terms. Where time restrictions call for a search with a high precision rate (i.e. with few irrelevant records), and where it is less important that all records are retrieved, then a search using index terms only (if such terms are available) can be conducted.

To view the thesaurus, click on MeSH Database link on the home page or the Advanced Search page then enter a term into the Search Box to identify any corresponding MeSH terms from the thesaurus. The methods used to build a search using MeSH terms are described in Step 4.

In other databases, to view the thesaurus it may be necessary to type the search term into the search box, 'turn on' a matching (mapping) facility by ticking the appropriate box, click on Search or Go and scroll down the displayed list to find relevant index term(s). It is usually possible to click on the index term to get an exact definition/description of that term. If a useful match for a concept is found, make a note of it, so it can be used in the search. Sometimes there will not be a convenient index term available, so stop searching if nothing is identified after looking up a number of different descriptions.

As well as helping to identify index terms of interest, a thesaurus can allow searching of a group of related index terms in one go. In this example, we are interested in non-pharmacological interventions for needle phobia. There are a number of indexing terms of interest listed in the thesaurus such as 'cognitive therapy', 'relaxation therapy', 'meditation', etc. Each of these terms could be added separately into a search strategy, but it would save time if all these related indexing terms could be added in one step. This is possible in many thesauri because index terms are listed in a hierarchy.

Basic structure of a thesaurus

A thesaurus orders index terms into hierarchical lists, with general terms at the top and more precise, specific terms underneath. These lists are often called tree structures (the lists 'branch out' rather like a tree). Figure 3.8 shows a section of a medical/healthcare thesaurus in PubMed. Terms at the top of a list are called 'broader terms' and those indented underneath are known as 'narrower' terms. In the example, 'relaxation therapy' is a broader term than 'meditation'; 'behavior therapy' is a broader term than 'relaxation therapy'; psychotherapy is a broader term than 'behavior therapy'.

Exploding index terms

To find articles indexed with the MeSH term 'behavior therapy', as well as articles indexed with the narrower MeSH terms such as 'relaxation therapy' and 'meditation', in one step, 'explode' the broader index term. PubMed defaults to the explode option so a search of a broader term will automatically retrieve articles that have been assigned 'narrower' MeSH terms. In other databases,

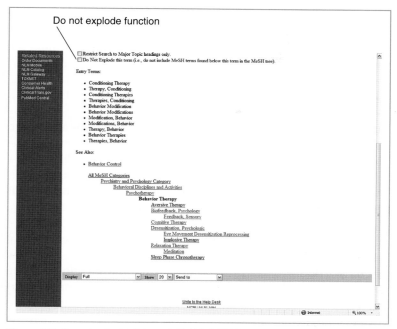

Figure 3.8 Example of a MeSH tree in PubMed (© National Library of Medicine, reproduced with permission.)

you may need to select and 'explode' button before pressing the 'search' button. In PubMed, exploding the index term 'behavior therapy' would automatically search the following index terms:

Behavior Therapy
  Aversive Therapy
  Biofeedback, Psychology
    Feedback, Sensory
  Cognitive Therapy
  Desensitisation, Psychologic
    Eye Movement Desensitisation Reprocessing
    Implosive Therapy
  Relaxation Therapy
    Meditation
  Sleep Phase Chronotherapy

The 'explode' function picks up everything *beneath and indented to the right* of the exploded term. You can choose to avoid this option by activating the 'Do not explode this term' button in the MeSH Database (Fig. 3.8).

Step 3: getting a search ready

Having checked through the details of the search tools and found some useful index terms to use, add that information into the written words/phrases list already prepared from the PICO question. It is a good idea to have a written plan of the search terms that will be typed into the search box, as well as the symbols that will be used. In this way, mistakes are less likely to be made.

The standard way of doing this is to write out the search as a series of steps, each step starting on a new line, with each new line being numbered. The final line of the search should bring together the combination of words you wish to find in the journal articles. This is also the standard format used for entering searches into a database. Box 3.4 shows a draft, hand-written search strategy comprising free text terms that we think represent the P and I components of our needle phobia question. In Box 3.5, we have further refined the proposed search strategy to include, in places, MeSH terms as opposed to free text

---

BOX 3.4 Draft search strategy for the question on needle phobia

#1   fear OR phobia OR anxiety OR stress

#2   needles OR syringes OR injections

#3   #1 AND #2

#4   cognitive behavioural therapy OR relaxation OR meditation OR meditate OR meditating OR desensitisation OR desensitise OR hypnosis OR hypnotherapy OR hypnotise OR coping skills OR relaxation

#5   distraction OR distracting OR distract OR diversion OR divert attention

#6   #4 OR #5

#7   #3 AND #6

BOX 3.5 Enhanced search strategy for the question on needle phobia, designed for PubMed: phrases are enclosed in double quotations; truncation (use with care) is indicated with an asterisk. Note, MeSH terms are used in preference to free text terms

#1   FEAR OR PHOBIC DISORDERS OR ANXIETY OR ANXIETY DISORDER OR STRESS, PSYCHOLOGICAL

#2   NEEDLES OR SYRINGES OR INJECTIONS OR BLOOD SPECIMEN COLLECTION

#3   #1 AND #2

#4   BEHAVIOR THERAPY

#5   hypnosis OR hypnotherapy OR hypnotise OR "coping skill*" OR "coping mechanism*" OR imagery

#6   distract*

#7   "divert attention" OR diversion

#8   #4 OR #5 OR #6 OR #7

#9   #3 AND #8

---

terms. This is to increase the precision of our search. We plan to use the exploded term 'behavior therapy', which will pick up articles that have been assigned the index terms relaxation therapy, meditation, etc. (as shown in Fig. 3.8). We have, therefore, deleted free text terms such as meditation, meditate, meditating, etc. In Box 3.5, the Boolean operators and the MeSH terms have been written in capital letters.

Step 4: entering your search strategy onto the database

At this point the search strategy is ready to be entered.

The first line of the written search strategy in the example (Box 3.5) comprises MeSH terms that have been identified from the thesaurus. Click on the MeSH Database link in the Advanced Search screen (link shown in Fig. 3.7) to access the MesH page (Fig. 3.9). Type the first term in the search box and click Go,

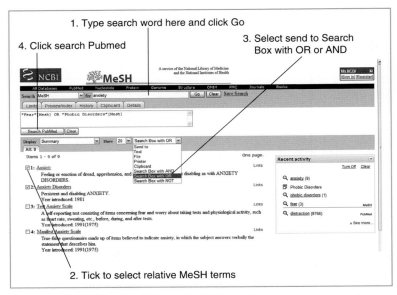

Figure 3.9 PubMed Mesh page (© National Library of Medicine, reproduced with permission.)

then select the appropriate MeSH term(s) from terms offered by ticking the relevant box(es). As previously stated, the default in PubMed is for the term to be exploded, so all index terms below the term selected will also be searched. Click Send to Search Box with AND or Send to Search Box with OR (depending on which Boolean operator is to be used), then, clear the search window (using Clear) and type the next search term to identify the MeSH term. Once all selected terms are in the search box, click Search PubMed. This will yield a list of references, all of which are indexed with one or more of the listed MeSH terms.

We want to add more lines from our written search to our search strategy so we ignore this list of references and click again on the Advanced search link. Continue building the search strategy: To add MeSH terms, follow the instructions above; to add free text terms, type each term into the blank search box then click Search. The database will look for any journal articles containing the words/phrases specified. Before entering the next search term, clear the search box using the Clear button next to the Search Box. This action does not lose the search: each line of the search will be retained. In PubMed it is possible to view exactly which terms the database has searched by clicking the Details link on the Advanced Search page. Figure 3.10 gives a list of terms searched when the truncated term distract* was typed into the Search Box. You can type the next line of the written search into the search box even if the Details page is open.

To view each line of the search (i.e. the search history) return to the Advanced Search page (Fig. 3.7) by clicking the Advanced search link. As shown, each line has automatically been assigned a number (#1, #2, etc.). Don't worry if, as in our search, the numbers do not start at #1 or are not consecutive. To combine the lines of the search, type the relevant line numbers, and the appropriate Boolean operators, into the search window. Continue building the search strategy to replicate, line by line (apart from the numbering), the written search plan. Figure 3.7 shows our completed search. #11 gives the final line of the P component of the search (1993 references were identified by this part of the search); #20 gives the final line of the I component of our search (89 027 references were identified by this part of the search). The overall final line of the search (in this example, line #21) brings together the journal articles that hopefully address the question. Our search identified 117 articles, some of which may be irrelevant. To view the identified references, click on the

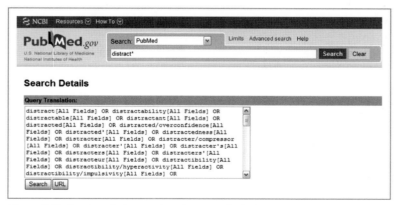

Figure 3.10 To view which terms have been searched when using a truncated search term, click on the Details link on the Advanced search page. (© National Library of Medicine, reproduced with permission.)

final line of the search in the Results column (Fig. 3.7). If you make a mistake (e.g. a spelling mistake) when searching for a term, just retype that search line, then when bringing together the lines of the search, exclude the incorrect lines. We excluded lines 16 and 18 from our final search line.

To restrict the retrieved references to, for example, English language articles and to studies conducted in humans only, click the Limits link and select the appropriate limits from the available options. By applying these limits to our search, the number of identified articles was reduced from 117 to 110. The Limits applied will be listed at the top of the results page to remind you that you have limited the search. To remove the limits (for example, to search additional terms for which the limits do not apply), simply click Remove on the Limits reminder.

Managing references

Depending on how many references are in that final group, they can be viewed and selected one by one on screen; but it is often preferable to download them onto your computer, ideally using software such as EndNote®, ProCite® or Reference Manager®. Software packages such as these have revolutionised the way in which references can be sorted and integrated into articles, dissertations and theses. There is no need to manually type and retype bibliography lists: bibliography lists are created with a few clicks of the button and are automatically re-ordered where appropriate. Time spent learning how to use a reference management package is time very well spent. In the absence of such software, references can be saved to a file on your computer as a word document. Look for the 'save/download' button to do this. There is usually the choice of which references to print/save and the specific fields to be included. In PubMed, click on the Display Settings link to select the required format. References can be displayed as shown in Figure 3.11 or, more helpfully, the abstracts can also be shown. Next, click the Send to link, and select File. You will then be asked where, on your computer, you would like to save the file.

This completes the procedure for doing a basic search on PubMed.

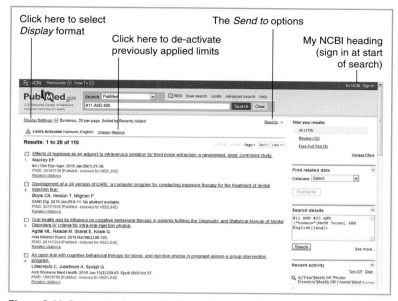

Figure 3.11 Retrieved references (© National Library of Medicine, reproduced with permission.)

Common queries regarding searching

In what order should search terms be typed up in a search strategy?

There are no strict rules on how a search should be typed out. Things can be done in any order; words/phrases can be split up so there are more lines in a search, or lumped together so there are fewer lines overall. As long as the logic of each step is correct and the final combination of words in the last line is correct, the result should be the same.

It is, however, advisable to search all the terms for one component of the question before starting on the next component. In this way, you will know whether or not it is necessary to add terms from a second or third component to the search. If a comprehensive list of search terms relating to the P component of your PICO question (combined with the appropriate Boolean operator) yields a manageable number of references, there is no need to add additional search terms from the I component of your PICO question. Indeed, it is advisable to only add search terms from a second or third component of the question if there is a need to further limit the number of references retrieved.

Is it better to use free text or controlled vocabulary (index terms)?

Which technique it is best to use depends on the search to be done. A search using index terms is more accurate because there is less need to think about all the different terminology that could be used to describe an illness or population, etc. Also, this approach limits the number of irrelevant articles identified. Where a database has controlled vocabulary for the topic of interest, it is best to use it. If a more thorough search is required, a combination of index terms and free text terms should be used (as index terms can be assigned incorrectly, or not assigned at all).

How do you know when all the relevant journal articles in a database have been found?

Unfortunately, there is no way to know if everything of interest has been found or not. Most bibliographic databases expand very quickly because so many journal papers are being published and added to the databases all the time. No one can keep track of precisely the subjects being covered. The idea of searching is to maximise the relevant articles that are found, whilst at the same time minimising the irrelevant material.

Finding 'most' of the useful information in a database is the best that can be hoped for. Searching is a pragmatic exercise and there is always the possibility that something will have been missed unintentionally, regardless of the experience of the searcher.

What do you do if you can't find any relevant articles?

This is often a problem when searching for evidence; there may be no references at all or items of poor quality only. In this situation it can be helpful to go 'back to the beginning' and look at the question and search strategy again. Devising a search strategy is a trial and error process and even experienced searchers will reconsider their approach a number of times if they struggle to find any useful results. It is not unusual for a 'final' search strategy to require a few attempts before it is generated.

There will be occasions, however, when in spite of trying a range of strategies or resources, no high-quality information is forthcoming and the best available evidence is expert opinion.

Tips for more advanced users

Proximity operators

Examples of proximity operators are WITH (used to find words/phrases contained in the same sentence), NEAR (used to find words/phrases contained in the same paragraph) and ADJ (used to find words that fall within a certain number of words of each other). The search 'midwife WITH care team' would find articles containing at least one sentence with both midwife and care team in it, and 'sickle cell NEAR leg ulcer' would find articles containing a paragraph with both sickle cell and leg ulcer in it. The search head ADJ2 neck' would find articles containing the words head and neck within two words of each other.

These sorts of tools are most useful in databases where the majority of records have an abstract or summary. Check the Help section to find out which proximity terms to use in a specific database.

Limiting to specific fields

Most database systems allow searches for information in the specific 'fields' of each journal article. This enables searches for words only in the title, articles by a specific author, or in a certain journal. Most systems tend to give each field in any article an abbreviated code, which can be used when searching. Check the 'help information' in a database to find out about the limiting options and how to select them.

To illustrate, in databases where the codes TI, AU, SO and AB are used to identify the fields Title, Author, Source and Abstract, the search 'injections[TI]' would find articles with the word 'injections' in the title field, 'Bloggs.au' would find articles with the word Bloggs in the author field, and 'nurse in SO' would find articles with the word nurse in the source field.

In PubMed, the search can be limited to a specific field either by adding the code (tag) using square brackets (for example, type 'Bloggs[AU]' in the search box) or by clicking the Limits tab on the features bar and selecting the appropriate Tag Term.

Subheadings

To help make an index term even more precise, or tailored to a specific aspect, some systems include an option to search an index term with certain subheadings attached. Subheadings are generally categories such as diagnosis, prevention, adverse reactions, complications, epidemiology, prognosis, surgery, etc. When an index term is assigned to an article, any appropriate subheadings will be linked to the term as well. If it is certain that the search only needs to focus on a narrow aspect of an index term, choosing the appropriate subheading(s) (rather than all of them) will limit the search to just the index term with that subheading attached. In PubMed, the subheadings can be viewed in the MeSH database (Fig. 3.12).

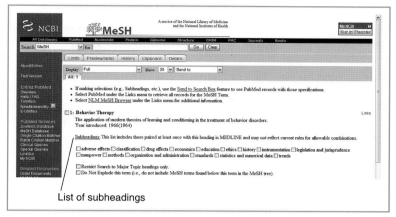

List of subheadings

Figure 3.12 Example of a MeSH heading and its Subheadings (© National Library of Medicine, reproduced with permission.)

Saving search strategies

Many database systems allow a completed search history to be saved, so the search can be run again, without having to type everything out all over again. Whilst this may not be a problem for short searches, once a search builds up a number of lines it can be very helpful to use this facility. In PubMed, the search history can be saved indefinitely using My NCBI. This requires that you sign into My NCBI before constructing the search. Check the 'help information' for more information.

Too many or too few articles

If too many articles are found it may be necessary to narrow down a search to make it more accurate. Use more precise index terms or link them to specific subheadings or perhaps search over a fewer number of years. It may be necessary to break up a broad subject into a series of questions, so the volume of information available can be better managed.

If only a few articles of interest are found, it may be necessary to widen out a search, so it is not so precise. Use broader index terms linked to all subheadings, or more general free text terms. If information is required on a very specific question, a low search result could mean little research has been done on that exact topic.

When to stop searching

This very much depends on the objectives of a search. If a comprehensive literature review is required, a number of different databases should be searched to get as much useful material as possible. If a few conflicting articles are required on a topic to get an 'evidence base' debate going or to stimulate discussion about treatment options, etc., a quick search on one database may be quite sufficient. If a good-quality, up-to-date evidence-based guideline, synopsis of evidence or a systematic review has been identified, searching may be stopped.

The amount of searching done will also be influenced by the resources that are available: the time and number of databases available. If comprehensive searches are done on a number of different databases, there will be gradually diminishing returns. The same journal articles will reappear each time and the volume of new articles identified will decrease. There will come a point when the effort involved in searching is not worth the tiny reward of new material found.

There is no right or wrong answer on when to stop searching. As with many aspects of the search process, it is a pragmatic decision. The main thing is to be explicit about which databases have been searched. This avoids any confusion and allows a search to be accurately updated or expanded by looking in different databases.

Searching for a systematic review

Undertaking the comprehensive searching required for a systematic review is not something that should be done lightly. It requires searching experience and knowledge of available resources. Teaching the skills for this type of searching is beyond the scope of this manual.

There is an increasing awareness that not all good-quality research work is published in professional journals; that much research is published in the form of conference proceedings, theses or project reports only; that many journals are not included in electronic databases; and that published research can be difficult to find, particularly where unexpected terminology has been used and/or index terms have not been assigned to articles. Systematic reviewers are charged with tracking down not only the easily accessible research, but also these more difficult to find studies.

Budgeting is necessary to ensure all searching-related activities (building comprehensive search strategies, accessing the appropriate databases, identifying hard-to-find studies, obtaining and translating articles) can be completed within the funding limitations.

Unpublished information and hand searching

If there is a journal that covers research relevant to a review but that is not included in the databases being searched, it may necessitate going through issues of the journal by hand. This sort of extra work cannot be done when time is restricted. However, the Cochrane Collaboration has a commitment to try and find unpublished RCTs by searching conference proceedings and by looking through journals by hand ('hand searching'). Any extra RCTs found in this way are published in the Cochrane Central Register of Controlled Trials on the Cochrane Library. This means that searching this database on the Cochrane Library provides a quick and practical solution for finding unpublished information for a review.

Research in progress

Systematic reviewers are also charged with identifying research that is in progress or about to be completed that could be relevant to the review. Much work is being done to encourage researchers to publish their research proposals. In the UK, the main repository for research proposals is the UK Clinical Research Network Study Portfolio from the National Institute for Health Research. It aims to contain details of government supported research in the NHS, to help keep track of what is going on and to avoid any unnecessary duplication. The equivalent resource for the US is ClinicalTrials.gov. from the US National Institutes of Health. There are also various lists appearing on the internet covering research in progress, such as the Current Controlled Trials site.

> The UK CRN Study Portfolio can be found at: http://public. ukcrn.org.uk/search/
>
> ClinicalTrials.gov can be found at: http://clinicaltrials.gov
>
> Current Controlled Trials can be found at: www.controlled-trials.com

Useful guides for systematic reviewers

- *Systematic Reviews CRD's Guidance for undertaking systematic reviews in healthcare,* 3rd edition 2009. Chapter 1, Section 1.3.1.: Identifying research evidence for systematic reviews; Appendix 2: Example search strategy to identify studies from electronic databases. www.york.ac.uk/inst/crd/systematic_reveiws_book.htm
- *Cochrane handbook for systematic reviews of interventions,* Version 5.1.0. Updated March 2011 (Chapter 6: Searching for Studies). Available on the internet: www.cochrane-handbook.org/ and also available on the Cochrane Library
- *Cochrane handbook for reviews of diagnostic test accuracy,* in progress April 2010 (Chapter 7: Searching for Studies). Available online: srdta.cochrane.org/handbook-dta-reviews and via the Cochrane Library
- NHS CRD Information Service – *Finding studies for systematic reviews: a checklist for researchers* (updated April 2008). www.york.ac.uk/inst/ crd/revs.htm

Practising your search skills

We hope the preceding sections have outlined the benefits of using a systematic approach when searching electronic databases. Box 3.6 is an aide memoir for the various aspects of searching that you may want to practise. We encourage you undertake the exercises provided (see website).

BOX 3.6 Key points to remember about searching electronic databases

1. Get help
   Attend training sessions in hospital/university libraries. Find out about support for searching in general.
2. Prepare the search
   Sort out the question/topic, generate word lists, have a draft search planned.
3. Find out more
   What database(s) might be useful to search, what tools they have (truncation, thesaurus, etc.), how those tools are used – check the 'help' information and any written guidelines.
4. Decide which database to search
   Plan so that you search resources in order of usefulness. Do a brief test search, check ease of searching, make sure all useful information is available.
5. Prepare the final search strategy
   Add in index terms, truncation symbols, etc. for the database to be searched.
6. Do the search
   Select index terms, type in free text terms. Get the final set of useful records at the end.
7. Print or save the final set of articles
   Print/save the records to look at later on.
8. Keep a record of the resources searched
   Make a note of the database, the version used (Ovid CD-ROM, SilverPlatter on the internet, etc.), the years searched and the date the search was done.
9. Keep a record of the search strategy
   Make sure a copy is kept, so the exact details are available for future reference.
10. If searching for systematic review, access sources of unpublished and ongoing research.

Summary

This chapter has provided an introduction on how to search the research literature to support evidence-based practice in healthcare. It has provided background on how databases of individual articles are organised and the basic principles that are used when searching for information on electronic systems. The use of a hierarchy of evidence for selecting resources to search first when trying to find answers to clinical questions has been highlighted. An example search on PubMed and some discussion of more advanced searching techniques has also been covered. The resources that are available to search will depend on local funding and access arrangements, so the importance of consulting the library services of which you are a member has been emphasised. It is important to remember that your library should be the first port of call to assist with searching questions and to provide hands on training sessions and individual support on the resources it provides and it may also be able to undertake searches for research evidence on your behalf.

References

DiCenso, A., Bayley, L., Haynes, B., 2009. Accessing pre-appraised evidence: fine-tuning the 5S model into a 6S model. Evid. Based Nurs. 12, 99–101.

Haynes, R.B., 2001. Of studies, syntheses, synopses and systems: the "4S" evolution of services for finding current best evidence. Evid. Based Med. 6, 36–38.

NHS CRD, 2001. Undertaking systematic reviews of research on effectiveness. CRD's guidance for those carrying out or commissioning reviews, second ed. CRD report number 4. Available online at: www.york.ac.uk/inst/crd/report4.htm.

Further reading

These are general articles about searching the healthcare literature aimed at the beginner/intermediate. As far as possible, they are directed at a nursing audience. They should give more advice and ideas on how to approach literature searching in the clinical setting.

Cooke, A., 1999. Quality of health and medical information on the internet. British Journal of Clinical Governance 4 (4), 155–160.

Cronin, P., Ryan, F., Coughlan, M., 2008. Undertaking a literature review: a step-by-step approach. Br. J. Nurs. 17 (1), 38–43.

Cullum, N., 2000. Users' guides to the nursing literature: an introduction. Evid. Based Nurs. 3, 71–72.

Ehrlich-Jones, L., O'Dwyer, L., Stevens, K., Deutsch, A., 2008. Searching the literature for evidence. Rehabil. Nurs. 33 (4), 163–169.

Glanville, J., Haines, M., Auston, I., 1998. Finding information on clinical effectiveness. Br. Med. J. 317, 200–203.

Hendry, C., Farley, A., 1998. Reviewing the literature: a guide for students. Nurs. Stand. 12 (44), 46–48.

Hunt, D.L., Haynes, R.B., Browman, G.P., 1998. Searching the medical literature for the best evidence to solve clinical questions. Ann. Oncol. 9 (4), 377–383.

Hunt, D.L., Jaeschhke, R., McKibbon, K.A., 2000. Users' guides to the medical literature: XXI using electronic health information resources in evidence-based practice. J. Am. Med. Assoc. 283 (14), 1875–1879.

Johnston, L., 2004. Research matters: searching for evidence to use in the practice setting. Neonatal, Paediatric and Child Health Nursing 7 (1), 26–28.

Lawrence, J.C., 2007. Techniques for searching the CINAHL database using the EBSCO interface. AORN J. 85 (4), 779–791.

Lowe, H.J., Barnett, G.O., 1994. Understanding and using the Medical Subject Headings (MeSH) vocabulary to perform literature searches. J. Am. Med. Assoc. 271 (14), 1103–1108.

McKibbon, K.A., Marks, S., 1998. Searching for the best evidence: part 1: where to look. Evid. Based Nurs. 1 (3), 68–69.

McKibbon, K.A., Marks, S., 1998. Searching for the best evidence: part 2: searching CINAHL and Medline. Evid. Based Nurs. 1 (4), 105–107.

NHS Centre for Reviews and Dissemination, 2001. Accessing the evidence on clinical effectiveness. Effectiveness Matters 5 (1). Available online at: www.york.ac.uk/inst/crd/em.htm.

Rau, J.L., 2004. Searching the literature and selecting the right references. Respir. Care 49 (10), 1242–1245.

Ringler, R.D., 2005. How to use the internet wisely. Nurs. Spectr. (Fla Ed) 15 (2), 26–27. Available online at: community. nursingspectrum.com/MagazineArticles/article.cfm?AID513487.

Sindhu, F., Dickson, R., 1997. The complexity of searching the literature. Int. J. Nurs. Pract. 3 (4), 211–217.

Sindhu, F., Dickson, R., 1997. Literature searching for systematic reviews. Nurs. Stand. 11 (41), 40–42.

Thomas, B.H., Ciliska, D., Dobbins, M., Micucci, S., 2004. A process for systematically reviewing the literature: providing the research evidence for public health nursing interventions. Worldviews Evid. Based Nurs. 1 (3), 176–184.

Thompson, C., 1999. Searching for the evidence. Nurs. Times/ Learning Curve 3 (3), 12–13.

Younger, P., 2004. Using the internet to conduct a literature search. Nurs. Stand. 19 (6), 45–51.

APPENDIX 3.1

Electronic databases

This is by no means a comprehensive list, but a selection that is most likely to be available on hospital or university computer networks.

General medical

MEDLINE	Produced by the National Library of Medicine (NLM) in the USA. Contains information from 1966 onwards. Uses index terms and has a thesaurus (MeSH). It has a USA and English language bias. Very widely available.
EMBASE	Produced by Elsevier Science, based in The Netherlands. Contains information from 1974 onwards. Uses index terms and a thesaurus (known as Emtree). Has a European bias and more emphasis on pharmaceutical information.

Nursing

CINAHL	Cumulative Index to Nursing and Allied Health Literature, produced in the USA. Contains information from 1982 onwards. Uses index terms and has a thesaurus (called the Subject Heading List). See website: www.cinahl.com
BNI	British Nursing Index, produced in the UK. Contains information from 1994 onwards. Consolidates, from 1994, the British Midwifery Index and Nursing Bibliography and RCN Nurse ROM. Has a UK and English language bias.

Specialist

AIDSLINE	Database of information on HIV and AIDS, produced by the NLM. Contains information from 1980 onwards.

CANCERLIT | Database of information on cancer, produced by the US National Cancer Institute.

CABHealth | Database of information relating to human nutrition; parasitic, communicable (including AIDS/HIV) and tropical diseases; medicinal plants and public health. Contains information from 1973 onwards. Strong international and developing country coverage. Uses index terms and has a thesaurus (CAB thesaurus).

AMED | Allied and Complementary Medicine, produced by the British Library. Contains information from 1985 onwards. Includes physiotherapy, occupational therapy, rehabilitation and palliative care. Uses index terms and a thesaurus (AMED thesaurus, based on MeSH).

PsycINFO | Produced by the American Psychological Association. Contains information from 1887 onwards. Covers all aspects of psychology. Uses index terms and a thesaurus (Thesaurus of Psychological Index Terms) for items dating from 1967 onwards.

LLBA | Linguistics and Language Behavior Abstracts. Contains information from 1981 onwards. Coverage includes speech, language and hearing pathology.

Health management

HealthSTAR | Produced by the NLM and American Hospitals Association (between 1978 and 1999). Contains information from 1975 onwards. Covers health-care planning, policy and administration. Includes effectiveness of procedures, products and services and evaluation of patient outcomes.

HMIC | Health Management Information Consortium database. Produced in the UK, an amalgamation of databases from the Nuffield Institute of Health (University of Leeds), the Department of Health and the King's Fund.

Others

EBM Reviews	Database comprising CDSR, DARE and the *American College of Physicians (ACP) Journal Club journal*.
Science Citation Index	Essentially an electronic version of the *Current Contents* publications covering scientific journals. Aims to add newly published articles on to the database promptly.
Social Science Citation Index	Sister publication to Science Citation Index, covering social science journals.

APPENDIX 3.2

Useful websites

National library sites

A first port of call for nurses employed by the NHS in the UK are the national library websites:

Health Information Resources from NHS Evidence:
http://www.evidence.nhs.uk/default.aspx

Health on the Net Northern Ireland (HONNI):
www.honni.qub.ac.uk/ElectronicResources/

The Knowledge Network from NHS Education for Scotland:
www.knowledge.scot.nhs.uk/home.aspx

Health of Wales Information Service, e-Library (HOWIS):
www.wales.nhs.uk/sites3/home.cfm?Orgid=520

These sites provide access to many of the organisations listed below.

Nursing organisations

For quality-assessed resources go to Intute's Nursing site:
www.intute.ac.uk/nmah

Royal College of Nursing: www.rcn.org.uk/

Royal College of Midwives: www.rcm.org.uk/

Nursing and Midwifery Council: www.nmc-uk.org/

Midwives Information and Resource Service (MIDIRS) – a 'not for profit' organisation: www.midirs.org/

Community Practitioners' and Health Visitors' Association:
www.unitetheunion.com/cphva

Evidence-based practice organisations

For a comprehensive list, go to 'Netting the Evidence – A ScHARR Introduction to Evidence Based Practice on the Internet':
www.shef.ac.uk/scharr/ir/netting/

Centre for Evidence Based Nursing:
www.york.ac.uk/healthsciences/centres/evidence/cebn.htm

Joanna Briggs Institute (Australia):
www.joannabriggs.edu.au/about/home.php

NHS Centre for Reviews and Dissemination (includes the publications *Effective Health Bulletins* and *Effectiveness Matters*):
www.york.ac.uk/inst/crd/

Cochrane Collaboration: www.cochrane.org/

Cochrane Library: www.thecochranelibrary.com/view/0/index.html

Cochrane Library User Guide for the internet:
www.thecochranelibrary.com/view/0/HowtoUse.html

Campbell Collaboration: www.campbellcollaboration.org/

Campbell Collaboration databases – C2 Library:
www.campbellcollaboration.org/Fralibrary.html

Clinical Evidence: www.clinicalevidence.com/ceweb/conditions/index.jsp

Health Evidence Bulletins Wales: www.hebw.cf.ac.uk

National Institute for Health and Clinical Excellence (NICE):
www.nice.org.uk/

NIHR (National Institute for Health Research) Health Technology Assessment Programme: www.hta.ac.uk

Health-care guidance and guidelines

Scottish Intercollegiate Guidelines Network: www.sign.ac.uk

National Institute for Health and Clinical Excellence: www.nice.org.uk

CKS: www.cks.nhs.uk/home

NLH Guidelines Finder: www.library.nhs.uk

National Guideline Clearinghouse (US guidelines): www.guideline.gov/

CHAPTER

Using evidence from qualitative studies

Bernie Carter and Lynne Goodacre

KEY POINTS

- Qualitative research is fundamentally interpretative; illuminating subjective meanings and committed to the expansion of knowledge through the partnership of the researcher and the participants.

- Qualitative research encompasses a range of different theoretical and methodological frameworks.

- The plurality of methodologies creates contested ground in terms of whether a single, standardised set of criteria can be applied to inform critical appraisal of qualitative studies.

- Qualitative research is based on the collection of word/text/ language and image-based data.

- Critical appraisal requires knowledge of different methodologies and methods and being able to make connections between the approaches used and claims made within a paper.

- Historically, evidence from qualitative research was placed lower in the hierarchy of evidence than quantitative research; this (as well as the notion of hierarchies) is now being challenged.

- In contrast, in quantitative research most appraisal tools or frameworks rely on a series of questions for a reader to pose linked to the processes of that research.

- Qualitative research can independently contribute to evidence as well as enhance quantitative research.

- Increasingly, mixed methods research (using both qualitative and quantitative approaches) is seen as contributing a sounder knowledge base for practice. However, no substantive systems for appraising mixed methods research exist.

Introduction

All scientific thinking is a mixture of quantitative and qualitative thinking...... Research is inquiry, deliberate study, a seeking to understand

(Stake 2010, p. 13)

This chapter focuses on qualitative research, its contribution to evidence-based practice, and how to appraise and use evidence from qualitative studies. Although rooted more firmly in social science than in medicine and health care, qualitative research is playing an increasing, albeit often times controversial role, in evidence-based practice. The term qualitative research encompasses a wide range of different research methodologies (Nelson 2008), but can broadly be described as being:

...concerned with the meanings people attach to their experiences of the social world and how they make sense of that world

(Pope & Mays 2006, p. 2)

It is this fundamental concern with meanings, experience and trying to understand how people make sense of their worlds that makes the contribution of qualitative research so potentially powerful. An evidence-based approach to practice that does not appreciate the meanings of things provides only a partial knowledge base from which to deliver health care. It is the concern with the 'subjective meaning of .... issues, events or practices' (Flick 2009, p. 472) that means that qualitative research contributes in a distinctive manner (Meadows-Oliver 2009) to the development of evidence and the development of practice.

Qualitative research is sometimes described in terms of how it differs from quantitative research (Grypdonck 2006). This is perhaps understandable as quantitative research is generally more familiar to practitioners searching for evidence to underpin their practice. However, this sets up the premise that research is binary: quantitative (solely focused on measurement and unable to contribute explanations about the social world) versus qualitative (solely focused on text, meanings and social experience). No such simple dichotomy exists. Meyrick (2006) proposes there are as many differences between different qualitative approaches as there are between qualitative and quantitative approaches.

The concept of what constitutes evidence (Rycroft-Malone et al 2004) is contested, as is the existence of hierarchies of evidence (Petticrew & Roberts 2003), which are said to be 'illusory' (Rawlins 2008, p. 2). Whilst qualitative research has been forced into a lowly position in the hierarchy of evidence (Rolfe & Gardner 2006), an emergence of interest in qualitative research means that it is acknowledged increasingly as a fundamental element of evidence-based practice. This interest has brought with it a concomitant demand for a structured appraisal method (or methods) to enable readers to determine the robustness of qualitative studies. This creates a challenge since, ideally, the appraisal method would cover the breadth of qualitative research rather than requiring a specific tool for each methodological approach.

Within this chapter we start by exploring 'what qualitative research is' through considering common characteristics and attributes. We overview the epistemologies, methodologies and methods used within qualitative research and explore the way that these, and the type of questions researchers ask, frame the research studies they carry out. We then examine some of the different approaches to appraising qualitative research and their contested nature. From there we guide the reader through an approach to appraising research which focuses on four key processes (epistemology, theoretical perspective, methodology and methods). Through this approach we explore the key issues underpinning each process and suggest suitable questions that a critical reader of a qualitative research paper should consider when trying to determine the robustness of the study. From this point, we move to acknowledge the increasing importance and emphasis placed on mixed methods research considering how this needs to be handled in terms of critical appraisal. Finally, we draw the chapter together by reviewing the key issues.

What is qualitative research?

Qualitative research 'primarily relies on human perception and understanding' (Stake 2010, p. 11) and is broadly interested in generating 'descriptions and situational interpretations of phenomena' (Stake 2010, p. 57) to add to our knowledge and understanding of phenomena. There are many different ways of describing qualitative research, some more complicated than others. Part of this complexity arises from the fact that qualitative research is not a unified field (Dixon-Woods et al 2004), encompassing as it does a range of different theoretical and methodological frameworks. This complexity has arisen because qualitative research has evolved within a number of different disciplines each of which has contributed to its development and shaped the way that it is presented. Avis (2005, p. 3) notes that as a consequence:

...almost every aspect of qualitative research.... ..... is the subject of controversy.

This controversy could be viewed as chaotic and problematic, but there is common ground. Many of the debates can be seen to be intrinsic to a research approach that has been absorbed within different disciplines and ways of thinking.

One way of trying to unravel the answer to the question – 'what is qualitative research?' – is to draw on Stake's (2010, pp. 15–16) six special characteristics of qualitative study:

1. Qualitative research is *interpretive* because it is predicated on the belief that people perceive things in different ways, attribute different meanings to things and construct meaning based on their understanding of things. Qualitative research accepts the notion of multiple realities or multiple points of view.

2. Qualitative research is *experiential, empirical and field oriented*; another term used to describe this is *naturalistic*. In this sense qualitative research is carried out in a natural setting (often described as the 'field') which is (usually) not manipulated, to try and explore how behaviours and opinions are expressed in the everyday world.

3. Qualitative research is *situational*. This links to the notion of research being experiential, naturalistic and based in multiple realities but extends the ways in which qualitative researchers accepts that life (and research) is influenced by the things that surround us. Qualitative research is oriented to *context* as it acknowledges that the things that surround us influence how we respond to situations and that such influences need to be taken into account if we are to understand them. What we know and how we know things changes depending on our experiences. There is a concern for the uniqueness of a particular setting and participants. The importance of context and the situational nature of qualitative research means that it is rare that it is designed to be generalisable, although good qualitative research aims to resonate with other situations, settings, experiences that have similarity to the one described.

4. Qualitative research is *personalistic* in that researchers value people's world views, aiming to understand individual perceptions. By 'following the data' and adopting an emic perspective (which considers 'the concerns and values recognized in the behaviour and language of the people being studied' (Stake 2010, p. 55)), the researcher aims to understand

issues of importance to the participants rather than those that researcher(s) might see as important.

5. Qualitative research should be **well triangulated** and **well informed**. Since qualitative research relies on interpretation, these interpretations need to be robust and built on solid data that the researcher has interrogated for alternative explanations. Although there are different types of triangulation (e.g. theoretical, methodological, methods, cases, investigator, data) it basically means that a conclusion is drawn from more than one source or perspective.

A well-reported study provides the reader with enough information to draw their own conclusions. Through the use of **reflexivity** within the study, and in the reporting of the study, the researcher's own particular position and other factors which could have influenced interpretation should be made clear.

6. Qualitative research is influenced by **strategic choices**. Some strategic choices are made at the start of the study and are guided by its underpinning purpose, for example, whether the purpose of the study is to contribute to policy development or a more general understanding of a situation or, whether it is aiming to contribute knowledge within a particular perspective, or aiming to change practice or uncover particular truths. Other strategic choices are made as the study progresses, for example, the question asked in an interview, or the people included in the sample.

To explore these six characteristics described by Stake (2010) in more detail it is perhaps worth considering an example drawn from an everyday situation, in this case a study about elderly people at risk from falls. The study itself would most likely draw on a population of elderly people who have fallen or who are at risk from falling and those who support and care for them. The following scenario might be typical of the population.

> After a minor fall an elderly man may perceive he is perfectly able to manage independently at home and is declining any professional support. His daughter may perceive that he is frail and unable to manage without some support but is concerned about eroding his independence so limits the amount of support she provides. Even in this simple example two views of the same situation are apparent. However, life rarely involves just the interaction between two

people. *In the situation described other people are likely to be involved each perceiving the situation from their own individual personal (and professional) perspectives. The neighbours may see the elderly man apparently struggling to cope and wonder why the daughter is 'doing so little'. The occupational therapist may perceive the risk of him falling as very high but be unable to intervene as he is declining all help. The perceptions of other members of the family, other friends, acquaintances and professionals will all be looking at the same situation, but perceiving things differently. Each person's perception will be influenced by who they are, what their role is, their previous experiences, what is at stake, and how they interpret the situation.*

The complexities of real-life situations such as these are ones which underpin and inform the way that qualitative research works and its potential contribution to the evidence base.

In the example above the qualitative researcher would need to engage with how the different people perceived the situation (*interpretive*) to be able to generate a knowledge base about the situation. The *experiential, empirical and field-oriented (naturalistic)* aspects of qualitative research could relate to a range of different settings (e.g. the man's home, the hospital, his community) or concentrate solely on one. The experiential focus results in an interpretative report constructed from what the researcher(s) has seen, heard and documented. In the example presented this interpretive approach would create greater insight into the situation that could help guide understanding and practice. Qualitative research does not aim to generate a complete understanding of an entire situation, but tends to focus on particular aspects so as to construct a deepened understanding of that aspect. For example, the dynamics between the daughter and her father could be explored to generate a deepened understanding of the meanings of the situation for them. This decision to focus on meaning could be one of a number of *strategic choices* made by the researcher throughout the study.

Acknowledging the *situational* aspect of this type of research and how *context* must be considered, we can see in the example above that the meaning of the situation changes as the situation itself changes. For example, if the fall the man has had is his first fall then the meanings are likely to be different to if it is his 50th fall; if he has needed to be hospitalised the meaning will be different to if he was able to get up without help; if his daughter finds him confused and lying on the floor then the meaning will be different to if he has telephoned her himself. Understanding context is fundamental to good qualitative research as without it the reported meanings will make less sense and be of less use as evidence.

For the research to remain *personalistic,* the researcher may have to lay aside their own professional perspective or personal values to try and understand, in the previous scenario, the perspective of the daughter, who appears angry.

In order to ensure that the findings are *well triangulated* and *well informed*, in the example referred to the evidence produced by the study should be a *reflexive* and detailed synthesis of the findings. This synthesis should create a clearer insight into the issues that underpin and inform the everyday situation of frail elderly people who have fallen or are at risk of falling.

Categorising qualitative research

Beyond these six characteristics there are generally two main approaches to describing qualitative research. The first adopts a more pragmatic approach describing qualitative research in terms of the data it aims to collect (mostly text/word and/or image based but not numerical data), the methods it uses to collect data (e.g. interviews, focus groups, diaries, photographs), and how it goes about analysing these data (e.g. through interpretation). The second is more philosophical and categorises qualitative research in accordance with the philosophical stance adopted by the researcher in framing their research question and how this then influences their approach to answering that question. The different approaches are informed by the researchers' beliefs about what 'exists' and 'constitutes social reality' (Blaikie 2010, p. 8). However, good qualitative research is generally a combination of clear and consistent philosophical decisions and choices about how to generate and analyse the data.

Four concepts underpin (explicitly or implicitly) almost any discussion about what qualitative research is; these are ontology, epistemology, methodology (the more philosophical elements) and methods (the more pragmatic element) (Table 4.1). These concepts also underpin quantitative research but tend to be more taken for granted; this is less so in qualitative research where they very clearly influence the direction, choices, design and outcomes of a study and the nature of the evidence generated.

Whilst these terms may seem a little obtuse there are good reasons for understanding the ontological and epistemological assumptions which underpin research. Grix (2002, p. 176) explains that they are needed in order to:

- understand the interrelationship of the key components of research (including methodology and methods);
- avoid confusion when discussing theoretical debates and approaches to social phenomena
- be able to recognise others', and defend our own, positions'.

Ontology is perhaps the most fundamental of these concepts as it relates to the assumptions and beliefs we hold about how the world is made up and the nature of things within the world. Barron (2006, p. 202) defines ontology as '*a concept concerned with the existence of, and relationship between different aspects of society, such as social actors, cultural norms and social structures*'. In qualitative research these beliefs need to be made explicit as they inform all choices made within a study, in particular which methodologies and methods are used. Understanding (or at least having a good basic grasp) of ontology is crucial to understanding qualitative research.

Table 4.1 provides an overview of definitions of terms and examples. We have chosen to draw on Crotty's (1998) definitions within this chapter; other writers present these ideas in different ways and with seemingly different emphasis (Blaikie 2010, Guba 1990). Crotty (1998) notes that separating ontology and epistemology can be difficult but we have presented this concept in the table as it is often referred to by authors within their reports.

TABLE 4.1 ELEMENTS UNDERPINNING AND INTRINSIC TO QUALITATIVE RESEARCH (DEVELOPED FROM CROTTY (1998))

Elements	Definition of term	Examples
Ontology	'the study of being. It is concerned with "what is", with the nature of existence, with the structure of reality as such' (Crotty 1998, p. 10)	
Epistemology	'the theory of knowledge embedded in the theoretical perspective and thereby in the methodology' (Crotty 1998, p. 3).	Subjectivism Constructionism
Theoretical Perspective	'the philosophical stance informing the methodology and thus providing a context for the process and grounding its logic and criteria' (Crotty 1998, p. 3).	Interpretivism (e.g. symbolic interactionism) Critical inquiry Feminism
Methodology	'the strategy, plan of action, process or design lying behind the choice and use of particular methods and linking the choice and use of methods to the desired outcomes' (Crotty 1998, p. 3).	Grounded theory Narrative inquiry Action research Discourse analysis Appreciative inquiry Ethnography Phenomenological research
Methods (of data generation)	'the techniques or procedures used to gather........ data related to some research question' (Crotty 1998, p. 3)	Interviews Diaries Focus groups Case studies Narratives Observation Photo-elicitation technique

TABLE 4.1 (CONTINUED)

Elements	Definition of term	Examples
Sources	the participants, places, settings and materials from which data are drawn in order to answer the research question in a way which is consistent with the methods, methodology, theoretical perspective and epistemology.	People (potentially taking into account gender, age, role, experience, diagnosis and other characteristics, etc.) Settings and environments (hospitals, clinics, surgeries, homes, hospices, etc.) Reports and records Media (newspapers, internet) Photographs, images, performances
Methods (of data analysis)	'the techniques or procedures used to .... analyse data related to some research question' (Crotty 1998, p. 3)	Thematic analysis Interpretative methods Documentary analysis Constant comparative method Framework analysis
Reporting	the ways in which qualitative research is reported and disseminated	Text (including reports, articles, narratives) Performance (video, drama, pictures, sculpting, dance)
Utilising and implementing	the ways in which qualitative research is utilised and implemented	As part of a mixed method study As a stand-alone study In a meta-synthesis Informing understanding, values and practice Contributing to policy & guidelines Shaping services Empowering service users and families

The role of qualitative research in evidence-based practice

There is now a wider acceptance that qualitative research has a role to play in evidence-based practice as ' [e]vidence-based health care is about applying the best available evidence to a specific clinical question' (DiCenso et al 1998, p. 39). Increasingly there is a sense that qualitative research can contribute – through a mixed methods approach – to the design of complex interventions (Hulscher et al 2006) and to randomised controlled trials (Schumacher et al 2005), although, arguably, the actual evidence for this contribution is less well explored (Corrrigan et al 2006, Lewin 2004). Some authors have claimed that qualitative research has had relatively little impact (Newman et al 2006) or that, despite obvious potential, 'qualitative research findings are scarcely used for tailoring and improving the design of interventions' (Jansen et al 2009, p. 225), whilst others discuss the ways in which qualitative research can contribute to 'expanding the boundaries of traditional empirical research and to improving patient care' (Lempp & Kingsley 2007).

However, in considering the contribution of qualitative research to evidence-based health care, Popay and Williams (1998) propose two models. The 'enhancement model', previously explored by other writers including Black (1994), focuses on the link to strengthening quantitative research evidence, whereas the 'difference model' suggests an independence from quantitative research and, therefore, an independent contribution to the evidence-base. Both models play a role in explaining the potential contribution of qualitative research to evidence-based practice. As qualitative research becomes more firmly embedded in healthcare research, its potential contributions are growing (see Box 4.1).

Appraising qualitative studies

Like Sandelowski & Barroso (2002, p. 10) we prefer 'the word *appraisal* as opposed to evaluation, as appraisal more explicitly encompasses understanding in addition to estimating value'.

BOX 4.1 Potential contributions of qualitative research to evidence-based practice

- Improving the accuracy and relevance of quantitative studies (Black 1994)
- Identifying appropriate variables to be studied in quantitative research (Black 1994)
- Explaining unexpected results from quantitative work (Black 1994)
- Generating hypotheses to be tested utilising quantitative methods (Black 1994)
- Exploring 'taken for granted practices' in healthcare and informing change to provide more appropriate/effective care (Popay & Williams 1998)
- Understanding factors that shape lay/clinical behaviour/developing 'interventions' (Popay & Williams 1998)
- Understanding patients' perceptions of quality/appropriateness (Popay & Williams 1998)
- Providing a better understanding of organizational culture and the management of change (Popay & Williams 1998)
- Informing evaluations on complex policy initiatives (Popay & Williams 1998)
- Providing 'important insights into the social values expressed by society as a whole' which should 'play a crucial role in shaping the decisions of bodies, like NICE, when advising on the use of interventions for whole healthcare' (Rawlins 2008, p. 32)
- Preparing for complex interventions by 'identifying and addressing barriers and facilitators to implementing the intervention' (Corrigan et al 2006)
- Impacting on patient care through 'understanding divergence' so that interactions can 'be changed and improved, leading to more effective processes and outcomes' (Ong & Richardson 2006, p. 370)
- Developing assessment tools that are grounded in the language, personal expectations and experiences of specific patient groups (McEwan et al 2004)

Central to the process of critical appraisal is ensuring that the appropriate questions are posed for the specific research study. There are ongoing debates about the way in which rigour should be assessed (Rolfe 2006), the terminology that should be used (Stige et al 2009) and the relative use of different appraisal frameworks (Bryman et al 2008).

Different approaches to appraising qualitative research

Many criteria and checklists have been developed to help readers appraise qualitative research. Indeed, Barbour (2001, p. 1115) notes that:

[c]hecklists have played an important role in conferring respectability on qualitative research and in convincing potential sceptics of its thoroughness.

However, a word of caution here; some checklists have been designed to be of most relevance to a particular type of qualitative research and, therefore, may have less value in guiding the appraisal of other approaches. The simple answer would seem to be to use a generic assessment tool that has less specificity, but that accommodates the breadth of qualitative research. However, as with many aspects of qualitative research, there is no clear consensus about what criteria should be used (Bryman et al 2008, Cohen & Crabtree 2008) or, indeed, if criteria which are often derived from quantitative discourses should be used at all (Eakin & Mykhalovskiy 2003).

Generic checklists are problematic (Stige et al 2009) as they are likely to miss the nuances of particular approaches and result in a less robust approach to appraisal. The CASP tool is a generic tool comprising a checklist of 10 questions (Public Health Resource Unit England 2006). Whilst this tool is clearly useful it is accompanied by a 'warning' that ' [i]t is *not a definitive guide* and extensive further reading is recommended' (emphasis in original) (Public Health Resource Unit England 2006, p. 1). Cohen and Crabtree's (2006) web-based review of different appraisal tools/criteria concludes that:

there cannot and should not be one set of criteria used to evaluate qualitative research

(Cohen & Crabtree 2006).

So.....which questions should be asked when appraising qualitative work?

In exploring the central role of the reader in the appraisal process Sandelowski and Barroso (2002, p. 10) describe appraisal as the *'exercise of wise judgement and keen insight in recognizing the nature and merits of a work'*. In this section we have sought to pose a number of questions to guide your appraisal and inform the judgements you make about the nature and merits of qualitative studies.

As we have already pointed out, qualitative research encompasses different theoretical and methodological approaches and, therefore, the questions you ask need to be specifically relevant. Critiques of qualitative studies will be flawed if inappropriate questions are asked. This can be a challenge to someone new to qualitative research as it requires a basic appreciation of what should ideally be happening epistemologically, theoretically, methodologically and in relation to methods (Cohen & Crabtree 2008). For example, unless you know something about the theoretical underpinning of phenomenology it will be difficult to critically appraise a phenomenological study.

We have structured this section to enable you to systematically and critically appraise a research paper in terms of its rigour and the transferability of the findings to your own clinical practice. We have given some guidance on how the questions may vary in studies using different theoretical approaches and in studies generating different kinds of data. Most good qualitative research papers, especially those published within healthcare journals, reflect a fairly standard structure and should feature the key elements previously presented in Table 4.1 (ontology, epistemology, theoretical perspective, methodology, methods of data generation, sources, methods of data analysis, reporting, and utilising and implementing). These elements are used as sections headings to help provide guidance about the sorts of questions you should be asking. However, making connections between what you read, the questions you ask and the answers you gain is also crucial (see Box 4.2).

> **BOX 4.2** Making connections
>
> Whilst we have provided examples of some of the key questions you should be asking as you read through a research paper, it is important to stress the importance within qualitative research of the connections and consistency between the different stages. Therefore, you need to use a broad lens to determine the consistency between each of the stages and a small lens to appraise the detail of each stage.

In essence, a critical appraisal of a qualitative study should be undertaken to establish the *trustworthiness* of a study. Lincoln and Guba (1985) propose four criteria to achieve this aim, and Seale (1999) suggests some ways in which these can be demonstrated (see Table 4.2).

Appraising epistemology

Popay and Williams (1998, p. 36) describe the 'primary marker' for qualitative studies as '*does the research illuminate the subjective meaning, actions and context of those being researched*'. Qualitative epistemology is grounded in **subjectivism** and **constructionism**. Therefore, one of the first questions relates to whether or not a qualitative approach was appropriate to answer the specific research question. This requires you to be able to identify a clearly articulated aim or research question and then to be convinced that a qualitative approach is relevant. If, for example, the aim of a study was 'to measure the impact on the quality of life of an intervention based on motivational interviewing for people with chronic pain, at six months from baseline, compared with conventional treatment' you would question the relevance of using a qualitative approach. On the other hand, if the stated aim was 'to develop an understanding of the experiences of people with chronic pain who have received motivational interviewing' then you would have more confidence that the right approach has been adopted.

TABLE 4.2 CRITERIA FOR JUDGING THE TRUSTWORTHINESS OF QUALITATIVE STUDIES

Criteria	Meaning (Lincoln & Guba 1985)	Some of the ways in which it can be established (Seale 1999)
Credibility	The extent to which the findings are credible	• Prolonged engagement in the process of data collection • The use of different (multiple) methods of data collection in the same study • Evidence of other people reviewing the findings during analysis • The search during data analysis for negative cases
Transferability	The extent to which the findings can be transferred to another context	• Accounts of participants and settings should be presented as detailed and rich descriptions to enable you to judge the transferability of the findings to other settings
Dependability	The extent to which the findings can be repeated if repeated with the same or similar subjects in the same or similar context	• Evidence of a process of audit taking place throughout the conduct of the study (including researcher reflexivity and potentially the use of others to audit the conduct of the study and process of data analysis)
Confirmability	The degree to which the findings are determined by the participants and not by the biases, motivations or perspectives of the researcher	• Evidence of reflexivity by the researcher of their role and influence in the study • Engagement of participants in stages of the analytical process

Epistemology: key appraisal questions
- Is the aim of the study articulated clearly?
- Is there a strong rationale for conducting a qualitative study?
- Has the rationale been made explicit in the aim of the study?
- Has the researcher stated their positioning within the study and demonstrated reflexivity?

Appraising the theoretical perspective

The theoretical perspective underpinning qualitative research has implications for every stage of the research process. Qualitative researchers do not take reality for granted, but see it as being constructed (that is, what people understand and believe to be real is based on their own and other people's experiences and ways of interpreting things) and relativistic (it is not fixed, is apprehendable and is driven by natural laws). The choice of theoretical perspective is strongly linked to the assumptions held by the researcher within the study about reality. Different theoretical perspectives, for example, interpretivism, critical inquiry and feminism, adopt different positions in terms of the stance they take in relation to reality and how this then effects the way that knowledge is created and the focus of research (Box 4.3).

Knowing whether a research study was informed by feminism or interpretivism or critical inquiry enables you to make the right connections and question, for example, whether a study that claimed to use critical inquiry had actually tried to challenge influences and bring about change.

Theoretical perspective: key appraisal questions
- Is there a clear statement of the theoretical stance which underpins the study?
- Is there an explanation of the relationship between the research question and the theoretical perspective adopted?
- Are the findings consistent with the theoretical perspective?

BOX 4.3 Three theoretical perspectives

- **Interpretivism** assumes that the social world is 'mediated through meaning and human agency; consequently the social researcher is concerned to explore and understand the social world using both the participants and the researchers understanding' (Ritchie & Lewis 2003, p. 17).

- **Critical inquiry** explores and challenges how social, political, cultural, economic or ethnic influences become integrated into social structures and influence experiences, behaviour and beliefs. A central tenet of critical inquiry is to challenge such influences and bring about change (Crotty 1998).

- **Feminism** is a theoretical perspective centring on the 'challenge to dominant assumptions, inequities and social injustice that relate to women. It is critical in the sense that it seeks transformation and emancipation. However feminism encompasses a diverse range of perspectives that reflect the many phases in its development' (Dykes 2004, p. 22).

Appraising methodology (and study design)

The terms methodology and study design are sometimes used interchangeably but are, in reality, two different things. Methodology describes the specific methodological framework within which the study was conducted. Study design provides a rationale for and description of how the study was conducted in terms of phases of data collection and choice of methods.

Methodology

A clear statement should be given about the methodological framework utilised, for example whether the study was ethnographic, narrative or action research (Box 4.4). Knowing this is crucial to the process of critical appraisal as this should determine the questions you might ask. The more you understand about a methodology, the more informed your decisions about rigour. So, an appreciative inquiry study that did not engage collaboratively

BOX 4.4 A brief overview of some key qualitative methodologies

- **Grounded theory:** 'The purpose of grounded theory is to develop new theoretical perspectives based on (or grounded in) people's actual experiences' (Fox et al 2007, p. 14). 'The interaction between data analysis, theory building and sampling is central to the development of grounded theory' (Harding 2006, p. 131).
- **Narrative inquiry:** 'The researcher explores the lives of individuals and the story of their lives. Narratives are seen as the stories that individuals tell about themselves to give order to their lives' (Fox et al 2007, p. 16).
- **Phenomenology:** '.... aims at gaining a deeper understanding of the nature or meaning of our everyday experiences. Phenomenology asks, "What is this or that kind of experience like?" ' (van Manen 1990, p. 9).
- **Ethnography:** '... is designed to analyse organisations, cultures or communities in their natural settings...The researcher tries to make sense of how these systems organise and operate' (Fox et al 2007, p. 14).
- **Case study:** 'An approach that uses in-depth investigation of one or more examples of a current social phenomenon, utilizing a variety of sources of data. A "case" can be an individual person, an event, or social activity, group, organization or institution' (Keddie 2006, p. 20).
- **Action research:** '...is a type of applied social research that aims to improve social situations through change interventions involving a process of collaboration between researchers and participants. The process is seen to be both educational and empowering' (Newton 2006, p. 2)
- **Appreciative inquiry:** AI, at its heart, is about studying and exploring what 'gives *life* to human systems *when they are at their best*' (emphasis added) (Carter 2006, p. 50) and (www.positivechange.org/appreciative_inquiry.html).
- **Discourse analysis:** '...looks at texts to explore the functions served by specific constructions at both the interpersonal and societal level' (Fox et al 2007, p. 13).

with participants, and focused solely on the problems in a clinic, would be at odds with the entire purpose of the study.

Study design

As suggested by Mason (2002, p. 4), the production of a definitive design set in concrete is impossible in qualitative research given its 'fluid, flexible, data driven and context sensitive nature'. You might be worried to read that the interview questions changed as the research progressed, or that the sample, rather than being pre-determined, was informed and guided by insights derived from ongoing analysis during data collection, however it may be appropriate that elements within a qualitative studies change as the study progresses. Rather than seeing such evolution as a limitation (as would be the case in a quantitative study), robustly described and explained changes should generally be perceived as evidence of the engagement of the researcher with the research process.

The stages of data collection and the methods of data collection should be clear and consistent with the theoretical approach adopted. You should be able to identify how many phases of data collection took place: was it, for example, a series of single interviews that took place during one time period, a series of interviews that took place at several time points or the use of interviews followed up with focus groups? The rationale for each data collection phase (if there was more than one) should be clear and there should be an explanation of why and when things took place and how the phases linked together.

Qualitative researchers use various methods of data collection (Box 4.5). There should be an indication of why each method of data collection was chosen. If more than one technique were utilised (multiple methods) this should be justified.

Clearly, good qualitative research design is contingent on a good ethical and moral stance being adopted by the researcher (Carter 2008) and diligent consideration of the risks to participants, settings and the researcher. Careful preparation of study design and study materials, adopting a reflexive perspective, identifying potential power relationships and ensuring that participants are respected, are ways of ensuring ethical and moral integrity within a qualitative study.

BOX 4.5 A brief overview of some key qualitative data collection methods

- **Observational research methods:** observation can be undertaken with the researcher adopting different roles ranging from participant observation where the researcher engages in the situation or setting to a more passive role where the researcher watches the behaviours and talk that occurs within the setting but does not become engaged.
- **Verbal research methods:** verbal methods include interviews (ranging from in-depth/focused interviews to semi-structured interviews), narratives, focus groups, small group discussions, activity oriented approaches and diaries.
- **Visual research methods:** visual methods draw on approaches such as photography, drawing, film, video, and performance.
- **Documentary materials:** documentary methods include newspapers, existing diaries, reports and records, media, autobiographies.

Although these four broad categories exist, there is often overlap. For example, observation requires the researcher to observe what is happening and to note what is said. Visual methods that generate drawings or photographs are often linked with discussion and exploration of the images. The context in which an interview takes place requires the researcher to make note of the setting and surroundings. An examination of diaries and newspaper reports may be linked to exploration of the similar stories from film.

The appraisal questions you ask in relation to methodology will help you to determine the **dependability** and the **credibility** of the study.

Methodology: key appraisal questions
- Has the methodological approach been stated?
- Is the design of the study consistent with the methodological approach?
- Is the design of the study clear in terms of what happens when?

- If the study has a number of phases of data collection, is each phase clear and has an explanation been given for the order in which the data are collected?
- Has a convincing rationale for the choice of method been provided?
- If the study uses multiple methods of data collection, has a clear explanation been given as to why the different methods are used and in what order they are used?
- Is the ethical stance adopted appropriate for the study? Have risks such as emotional harm or distress been addressed.
- Is there evidence of reflexivity in relation to ethical and moral issues?

Appraising methods of data collection and sources of data

The most common methods of data collection used in qualitative research can be divided into four categories based around observation, verbal methods, visual methods and existing documents and materials (Box 4.5). The key focus of your attention in appraising this element of a study should be on their relevance to the research question and methodological framework, and the clarity and level of detail with which the methods are described. The most commonly used methods are interviews, focus groups and observation although visual methods are increasing in prominence.

Relevance to methodological stance

The methods used should be consistent with the specific methodological framework within which the study was located: if a phenomenological study aims to ask, 'What is this or that kind of experience like?' (van Manen, 1990, p. 9), the methods of data collection should reflect this aim; if postal questionnaires comprised mainly of closed questions were utilised, you might question the depth of detail obtained and the **credibility** of the findings; if a researcher described conducting an observational study based on a single episode of observation, similar concerns should be raised. The detail provided about the methods should enable you to answer some of the questions in Table 4.3.

Methods of data generation: key appraisal questions
- Are the methods consistent with the theoretical and methodological approach adopted in the study?
- Are the methods appropriate to the aim of the study?
- Are the methods described clearly?
- Is it clear how the data were collected?
- If there have been changes in techniques or focus have these been clearly articulated and are these reasonable?
- Is the period of engagement in data collection enough to convince you that the findings are credible?

Appraising sampling and recruitment

A sample may comprise, amongst other things, people, settings, environments, organisations, documents, the internet or visual material. Conscious choices will have been made regarding the population from which the sample was drawn, the size and relevant characteristics or features. In critically appraising a study, questions should focus on why and how these decisions were made, the impact that the sample had on the results and the implications in terms of the **transferability** of the findings to other contexts. A number of approaches to sampling are used, the most common of which are purposive, theoretical and convenience sampling (Box 4.6).

In critiquing samples for qualitative studies people often focus on the size of the sample which, whilst important, detracts from equally important questions about its characteristics and composition. To illustrate this point, qualitative research may be used to identify potential items to include in patient reported outcome measures. If the sample comprised only men who had been living with impairment for a year, you may question the utility of the outcome measure if used with women who had been living with the impairment for over 10 years.

The focus on the size of a sample may be due to the fact that many researchers may just state a number and leave you wondering how it was arrived at. You should be able to understand the decisions and choices informing the size of the sample, and

TABLE 4.3 FACTORS TO CONSIDER IN RELATION TO METHODS

Question	Examples
What method(s) was used?	It should be clear whether data were collected via single or multiple methods. It is common in qualitative research for a number of different methods to be used in a single study. An observational study may include observation, interviews with key informants and examination of documents and texts.
How was the method used?	The way in which methods are used will vary. Interviews and focus groups may be semi-structured and guided by a schedule or adopt a more open narrative approach in which a single question is posed to stimulate discussion. Observation may be conducted as a participant involved in the processes being observed or as a non-participant in a less engaged way. The description of the chosen method should enable you to understand clearly what was done and how; it should be congruent with the aim of the study, the methodology and theoretical perspective.
Where did data collection take place?	A characteristic of qualitative research is that it is naturalistic. However, it is carried out in a range of settings which have the potential to influence the information obtained. For example, if a study exploring compliance with treatment took place in the clinical setting where treatment was provided, this may influence what participants felt able to say.
Who was involved in data collection and if multiple people how was consistency assured?	An indication should be given of who was involved in data collection. For example, if a study not only took place in a clinical setting but was conducted by the person responsible for providing the treatment then even more concerns should be raised relating to the *credibility* of the findings. If several researchers were involved in collecting data they may be collecting it in different ways or asking totally different questions. You might want to explore how a degree of consistency was maintained.
How long did data collection last and was the duration of engagement commensurate with the aims of the study	In returning to Lincoln and Guba's (1985) criteria for assessing the trustworthiness of a study *credibility* is enhanced by prolonged engagement in the field. Phenomenological and ethnographic studies aim to elicit rich and deep insights. If interviews were conducted that only lasted 20 minutes or a single observation was undertaken, you might question the depth of insight obtained.

BOX 4.6 A brief overview of some key sampling approaches

- **Purposive sampling** occurs when participants, settings or documents are selected because they have specific characteristics or features which will enhance understanding of the research topic (Ritchie & Lewis 2003). These are identified prior to the commencement of the study and monitored as the recruitment progresses. You should be able to identify clearly the characteristics chosen and determine their relevance to the aim of the study and any impact they may have on its transferability.

- **Theoretical sampling** is often associated with grounded theory as the sample evolves during data collection. An initial sample will be selected and a period of data collection and analysis undertaken. A further sample is then determined informed by the analysis of the first data set. This process continues until 'data saturation', the point at which no new insights are obtained, is reached (Ritchie & Lewis 2003). In critiquing this approach you need to see that data collection, analysis and recruitment occurred as an iterative process and be convinced that data saturation was reached.

- **Convenience sampling** occurs when a researcher chooses a sample because it is easy to access. It is important to look at the influence this will have on the data collected. A researcher may recruit participants from their own caseload or colleagues with whom they work and therefore their relationship with participants may influence the information provided or the questions a researcher may have felt able to ask. Recruiting in this way is not necessarily wrong but you should (a) be aware of the potential impact of this decision on the data generated and (b) be reassured that the researcher has taken account of and tried to minimise any potential impact this may have had.

---

assess for yourself how this may have impacted on the data generated.

The **transferability** of the study can be assessed by the level of description given about the sample. To say that an observational study was conducted 'in a busy out-patient clinic' tells you little *about* the setting, or saying that 'eight women took part in the study' tells you nothing *about* the women. The researcher should enable you to understand who was involved in the generation of the data.

If a sample comprises people, the process of recruitment should be clear, enabling you to assess any impact this may have had on who took part in the study.

Sampling: key appraisal questions
- Is the population from which participants were drawn stated clearly?
- Is there an explanation of the way in which the sample was identified?
- Is the sample relevant to the aims of the study?
- Were specific characteristics sought in the sample and if so is the rationale for this explained?
- Is there a justification for the size of the sample?
- Does the sample enhance or limit the transferability of the findings to other contexts?
- Did the process of recruitment influence the composition of the sample?
- If the sample is part of a practitioner's caseload, are the rationale and safeguards for this clearly stated?

Appraising methods of analysis

The way in which analysis is undertaken within qualitative studies can sit uncomfortably with people who are used to a more quantitative approach. Interpretation built on the researcher's iterative exploration of the data is fundamental to qualitative research. Rigorous qualitative work does not simply report or describe what the researcher has gained from their data, but it goes beyond this to a deeper conceptual engagement. Returning to Stake's characteristics, the analysis should be interpretive, situated, oriented to context, personalistic, highly reflexive, and emic.

In terms of evidence of depth of analysis, you need to question if the analysis moves through an analytical hierarchy (Ritchie & Lewis 2003) from phases of data management (assigning codes and reorganising data under codes), to describing the data using illustrative quotes or examples, to an interpretation of the meaning and significance. For example, a results section may identify that five themes were created and may provide a description of each theme, illustrated with in-text quotes but you may be left asking yourself 'so what' because the author has not gone on to interpret their meaning.

Lincoln and Guba (1985) propose that researchers should provide evidence of an audit trail throughout the analysis to enable someone else to gain insight into the process and decisions that were made. Whilst comprehensive access to this audit trail will not be available to the reader, normally reference to this should be made in the paper. Different approaches to analysis can be adopted (Box 4.7).

There are a number of things which can be undertaken to increase the credibility and trustworthiness of the analysis (Box 4.8).

Methods of data analysis: key appraisal questions

- Is the approach to analysis explained clearly?
- Is the description of the choices made by the researcher clear in relation to coding and development of categories/themes/patterns?
- Is it possible to understand the different stages of the process and how they were undertaken?
- If multiple methods of data collection were used is there an explanation of how they are combined in the process of analysis?
- Is there a robust presentation of how deviant/negative cases were handled?
- Is it clear that alternative explanations were sought and taken-for-granted assumptions were challenged?
- Are the findings presented plausible?
- Would someone in the same situation/setting recognise what was being presented?
- Has the researcher tried to account for tacit (implicit) knowledge?
- If participant validation/member checking has been used, is this evident and is there evidence of responsiveness to this?
- Do the quotations and other sources of evidence provide a robust and sufficient base from which the claims are made?
- Are the inferences logical?
- Is there sufficient detail provided so that the reader can follow the interpretation and analysis?

BOX 4.7 A brief overview of analytical approaches

- **Thematic analysis:** 'is an approach that draws codes into groups, the groups into sub-themes, the sub-themes into themes and then the themes into a global theme that pulls everything together' (Carter 2004, p. 91).
- **Grounded theory analysis:** this is an inductive approach to analysis in which data collection, analysis and theory development are inter-related. The analysis process encompasses open, axial and selective coding which is undertaken to inform the development of a substantive theory (Strauss & Corbin 1990).
- **Framework analysis:** developed at the National Centre for Social Research utilises a thematic framework to classify and organise data according to key themes and concepts which evolve during familiarisation with the data. These are then charted within a matrix or table to inform the development of descriptive and explanatory account (Ritchie & Lewis 2003).
- **Narrative analysis:** focuses on the identification of key stories within the data and the meaning of the story, the way it is constructed and the intention of the storyteller (Riessman 1993).

BOX 4.8 A brief overview of approaches to credibility and trustworthiness in data analysis

- **Member checking** (validation): provides the opportunity for the people involved in the generation of the data to review it and to explore their agreement (or not) with the way in which they are being represented (Seale 1999). The whole transcript of a summary of an interview may be returned to participants for comment.
- **Search for negative cases:** Lincoln and Guba (1985) propose the search for negative cases as a way of increasing the credibility of analysis. This requires a researcher to explore and report upon situations when experiences or points of view may not always be consistent amongst all participants.
- **Triangulation:** is the '"process by which the phenomenon of topic under study is examined from different perspectives... findings of one type of method (or data, researcher, theory) can be checked out by reference to another'" (Holloway & Wheeler 2010, p. 308).

Appraising the reporting of the study

Virtually the whole of this chapter is devoted to appraising the reporting of qualitative studies. There is 'no one style for reporting the findings from qualitative research' (Sandelowski 1998, p. 376). The process of publication constrains the depth of description and the breadth of discussion of philosophical issues. Even the most diligent researcher who has completed a very rigorous study faces some fundamental choices about what to include and what to leave out of an article. These choices are forced on them by journal style guidelines and by word length. Some journals have more flexible style guidelines and more generous word counts but many constrain the reporting of qualitative research. Other choices made by qualitative researchers include the language they use and how theoretical they are in presenting their ideas. Sandelowski (1998, p. 375) makes us smile when she describes the offences to good writing that some qualitative researchers make, including the use of:

> *turgid prose, seemingly endless lists of unlinked codes and categories, dangling participles, and dizzying arrays of multiply hyphenated and, sometimes, nonexistent words that convey nothing more than the writer's willingness (albeit unintended) to destroy the English language.*

Clearly this is to be avoided. Wolcott (2002, p. 102) provides guidance that qualitative researchers should 'strive for more candor, to be straightforward in what we report and how we link up with the work of others'. Gilgun (2005, p. 260) makes an eloquent plea for the use of 'evocative, compelling writing' and 'lively, first-person, multiple-voiced texts' as a means of avoiding silencing the voice of the participants and researcher.

The researcher should demonstrate the connections between the various elements of their research within their writing.

Reporting: key appraisal questions

- Has the researcher clearly reported the study using a method appropriate to the epistemological and methodological stance?
- Has the researcher demonstrated engagement and collaboration with participants (as appropriate) in the report
- Is the writing accessible to the intended audience?
- Has the researcher been sufficiently reflexive in their engagement throughout the study?
- Have they clearly positioned themselves within the study?
- Has the researcher become too close to the participants?
- Has the researcher accounted for researcher bias (e.g. unexplored data in the field notes, feelings of empathy for participants swaying the presentation of findings)?
- Are any claims for generalisabilty supported, justified and reasonable?
- Is there evidence that the researcher has been flexible in the conduct of the study? Are any changes to design reported clearly?
- Is the reporting of the study accurate and unexaggerated?
- Is the value and importance of the study clearly presented?
- Is it clear how the study contributes to the body of knowledge in the topic area/disciplinary field/practice setting?
- Is the writing engaging and evocative?
- Has the researcher used the first person and demonstrated evidence of participants' voices?

Mixed methods research

The use of mixed methods research is increasingly common in health research. A clear distinction should be made between multiple methods research (using different methods of data collection from the same epistemological stance) and mixed methods (combining elements of quantitative and qualitative approaches within the same study) (Johnson et al 2007). Central to the use of mixed methods is the belief that using both approaches together has the potential to provide a better understanding than if either were used on their own (Creswell & Plano Clark 2007) (Box 4.9). Methods can be mixed in a number of different ways and Johnson

BOX 4.9 A brief overview of four different approaches to mixed methods design (Creswell & Plano Clark 2007)

- **Triangulation design:** concurrent collection of quantitative and qualitative data which are analysed separately and merged during interpretation
- **Embedded design:** one approach is given dominance and the other plays a secondary role. An example may be a smaller qualitative study embedded with a randomised control trial. But the two approaches are linked
- **Explanatory design:** a two phase design with data being collected at different times. Often qualitative data are used to explain quantitative findings
- **Exploratory design:** a two phase design, but the qualitative data collection comes first and plays the primary role in interpretation

et al (2007) position them on a continuum in which different or equal weighting is given to each component (Fig. 4.1).

Mixed method studies should demonstrate rigour within both the quantitative and qualitative phases and reports should provide answers to some additional questions about how the methods were mixed in the different stages of the research process: design; data collection; data analysis, and the weighting given to each.

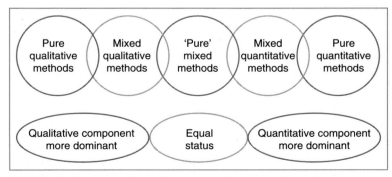

FIGURE 4.1 Continuum of research designs: qualitative through mixed methods to quantitative

TABLE 4.4 APPROACHES TO MIXED METHODS SAMPLING (DEVELOPED FROM ONWUEGBUZIE & COLLINS 2007)

Approach	Definition	Example
Identical	the same sample members participate in the quantitative and qualitative phases	The same patients with heart failure who completed a questionnaire about the frequency and extent of their symptoms also contribute through in-depth interviews about how their symptoms make them feel
Parallel	the sample participating in each phase is different but drawn from the same overall population	Boys aged 7–11 years old requiring post-operative pain management after orthopaedic surgery are recruited to the study. In hospital A, they complete the survey (Phase 1) and in Hospital B they participate in the interviews (Phase 2).
Nested	the same sample with a subset being chosen for the nested component	After contributing to a Quality of Life (QoL) questionnaire a smaller group of carers representing the highest and lowest QoL scores are asked to maintain narrative diaries of their experiences of caring for their spouse
Multilevel	the sample is drawn from different levels of the study population	Expert opinion is sought via Delphi technique from health care professionals about the management of violence and aggression on a Dementia Care Unit; subsequently the perspectives of patients and relatives are sought about the issue.

Sampling is central to a mixed methods study, and Onwuegbuzie and Collins (2007) have described four approaches (Table 4.4).

Although more mixed method studies are being undertaken, their conduct is not without challenges as rigour has to be demonstrated within each phase of data collection and information provided about how the methods were mixed and integrated. There are no substantive systems for appraising mixed methods research (Pluye et al 2009).

Conclusion

Good qualitative research is thorough, reliable, rigorous, explanatory, transparent, reflexive and, according to Brown (2010), undertaken by informed and confident researchers. Many of these same attributes are required by people appraising qualitative research. Reading qualitative research will require you to consider the choices and decisions made by the researcher, the consistency between all elements of the study and the fit with the findings. Appraising qualitative research requires the reader to be open to the interpretations presented by the researcher whilst maintaining a critical stance.

We have proposed a series of questions that could be posed (Box 4.10). Not every question is suitable for every type of qualitative study. Indeed, if a reader posed every question they would tie themselves in knots and appraising a paper would take an eternity. Making an informed selection from the proposed questions is a good way forward, although appraisers with less experience of qualitative research may find this challenging. For this reason, standardised checklists that may help to identify problem areas as well as the strengths of a qualitative study have been proposed. However, this guidance should not be so constraining that good qualitative research is strangled by a reductionist checklist and discarded. Good qualitative studies need room to breathe so as to inform practice with rich, subjective, meaningful and people-oriented evidence.

Exercise

We encourage you to consolidate your learning by undertaking the worked exercise on the website.

BOX 4.10 An overview of key questions to consider asking when appraising a qualitative study

Epistemology
- Is the aim of the study articulated clearly?
- Is there a strong rationale for conducting a qualitative study?
- Has the rationale made explicit in the aim of the study?
- Has the researcher stated their positioning within the study and demonstrated reflexivity?

Theoretical perspective
- Is there a clear statement of the theoretical stance which underpins the study?
- Is there an explanation of the relationship between the research question and the theoretical perspective adopted?
- Are the findings consistent with the theoretical perspective?

Methodology
- Has the methodological approach been stated?
- Is the design of the study consistent with the methodological approach?
- Is the design of the study clear in terms of what happens when?
- If the study has a number of phases of data collection is each phase clear and has an explanation been given for the order in which the data are collected?
- Has a convincing rationale for the choice of method been provided?
- If the study uses multiple methods of data collection has a clear explanation been given as to why the different methods are used and in what order they are used?
- Is the ethical stance adopted appropriate for the study? Have risks such as emotional harm or distress been addressed.
- Is there evidence of reflexivity in relation to ethical and moral issues?

Methods of data generation
- Are the methods consistent with the theoretical and methodological approach adopted in the study?
- Are the methods appropriate to the aim of the study?
- Are the methods described clearly?
- Is it clear how the data were collected?

(Continued)

BOX 4.10 An overview of key questions to consider asking when appraising a qualitative study—Cont'd

- If there have been changes in techniques or focus have these been clearly articulated and are these reasonable?
- Is the period of engagement in data collection enough to convince you that the findings are credible?

Sampling
- Is the population from which participants were drawn stated clearly?
- Is there an explanation of the way in which the sample was identified?
- Is the sample relevant to the aims of the study?
- Were specific characteristics sought in the sample and if so is the rationale for this explained?
- Is there a justification for the size of the sample?
- Does the sample enhance or limit the transferability of the findings to other contexts?
- Did the process of recruitment influence the composition of the sample?
- If the sample is part of a practitioner's caseload are the rationale and safeguards for this clearly stated?

Methods of data analysis
- Is the approach to analysis explained clearly?
- Is the description of the choices made by the researcher clear in relation to coding and development of categories/themes/patterns?
- Is it possible to understand the different stages of the process and how they were undertaken?
- If multiple methods of data collection were used is there an explanation of how they were combined in the process of analysis?
- Is there a robust presentation of how deviant/negative cases were handled?
- Is it clear that alternative explanations were sought and taken-for-granted assumptions were challenged?
- Are the findings presented plausible?
- Would someone in the same situation/setting recognise what was being presented?
- Has the researcher tried to account for tacit (implicit) knowledge?
- If participant validation/member checking has been used, is this evident and is there evidence of responsiveness to this?
- Do the quotations and other sources evidence provide a robust and sufficient base from which the claims are made?

BOX 4.10 An overview of key questions to consider asking when appraising a qualitative study—Cont'd

---

- Are the inferences logical?
- Is there sufficient detail provided so that the reader can follow the interpretation and analysis?

Reporting
- Has the researcher clearly reported the study using a method appropriate to the epistemological and methodological stance?
- Has the researcher demonstrated engagement and collaboration with participants (as appropriate) in the report?
- Is the writing accessible to the intended audience?
- Has the researcher been sufficiently reflexive in their engagement throughout the study?
- Have they clearly positioned themselves within the study?
- Has the researcher become too close to the participants?
- Has the researcher accounted for researcher bias (e.g. unexplored data in the field notes, feelings of empathy for participants swaying the way presentation of findings)?
- Are any claims for generalisabilty supported, justified and reasonable?
- Is there evidence that the researcher has been flexible in the conduct of the study? Are any changes to design reported clearly?
- Is the reporting of the study accurate and unexaggerated?
- Is the value and importance of the study clearly presented?
- Is it clear how the study contributes to the body of knowledge in the topic area/disciplinary field/practice setting?
- Is the writing engaging and evocative?
- Has the researcher used the first person and demonstrated evidence of participants' voices?

References

Avis, M., 2005. Is there an epistemology for qualitative research? In: Holloway, I. (Ed.), Qualitative research in health care. Open University Press, Maidenhead, pp. 3–16.

Barbour, R.S., 2001. Checklists for improving rigour in qualitative research: the case of the tail wagging the dog? Br. Med. J. 322, 1115–1117.

Barron, L., 2006. Ontology. In: Jupp, V. (Ed.), The sage dictionary of social research methods. Sage Publications Ltd, London, pp. 202–203.

Black, N., 1994. Why we need qualitative research. J. Epidemiol. Community Health 48 (5), 425–426.

Blaikie, N., 2010. Designing social research, second ed. Polity Press, Cambridge.

Brown, A.P., 2010. Qualitative method and compromise in applied social research. Qualitative Research 10 (2), 229–248.

Bryman, A., Becker, S., Sempik, J., 2008. Quality criteria for quantitative, qualitative and mixed methods research: a view from social policy. Int. J. Soc. Res. Methodol. 11 (4), 261–276.

Carter, B. 2006, "'One expertise among many'– working appreciatively to make miracles instead of finding problems: Using appreciative inquiry as a way of reframing research", Journal of Research in Nursing,vol. 11, no. 1, pp. 48–63.

Carter, B., 2008. 'Good' and 'bad' stories: decisive moments, 'shock and awe' and being moral. J. Clin. Nurs. 17, 1063–1070.

Cohen, D., Crabtree, B., 2006. Using qualitative methods in healthcare research. A comprehensive guide for designing, writing, reviewing and reporting qualitative research. Qualitative Research Guidelines Project. Robert Wood Johnson Foundation, Princeton, NJ. http://www.qualres.org/ Date last accessed 28/03/2011.

Cohen, D.J., Crabtree, B.F., 2008. Evaluative Criteria for Qualitative Research in Health Care: Controversies and Recommendations. Ann. Fam. Med. 6 (4), 331–339.

Corrrigan, M., Cupples, M., Smith, S., Byrne, M., Leathem, C., Clerkin, P., et al., 2006. The contribution of qualitative research in designing a complex intervention for secondary prevention of coronary heart disease in two different healthcare systems. BMC Health Serv. Res. 6 (1), 90.

Creswell, J.W., Plano Clark, V.L., 2007. Designing and conducting mixed methods research. Sage Publications Ltd, Thousand Oaks.

Crotty, M., 1998. Foundations of social research: meaning and perspective in the research process. Sage Publications, London.

DiCenso, A., Cullum, N., Ciliska, D., 1998. Implementing evidence-based nursing: some misconceptions. Evid. Based Nurs. 1 (2), 38–39.

Dixon-Woods, M., Shaw, R.L., Agarwal, S., Smith, J.A., 2004. The problem of appraising qualitative research. Qual. Saf. Health Care 13 (3), 223–225.

Dykes, F, (2004) What are the foundations of qualitative research? In: Lavender T, Edwards G and Alfiric Z (eds) Demystifying Qualitative research: A resource book for Midwives and Obstetricians. London: Quay Books.

Eakin, J.M., Mykhalovskiy, E., 2003. Reframing the evaluation of qualitative health research: Reflections on a review of appraisal guidelines in the health sciences. J. Eval. Clin. Pract. 9 (2), 187–194.

Flick, U., 2009. An introduction to qualitative research. Sage Publications Ltd, London.

Fox, M., Martin, P., & Green, G., 2007. Doing Practitioner Research Sage Publications, London.

Gilgun, J.F., 2005. "Grab" and good science: Writing up the results of qualitative research. Qual. Health Res. 15 (2), 256–262.

Grix, J., 2002. Introducing students to the generic terminology of social research. Politics 22 (3), 175–186.

Grypdonck, M.H., 2006. Qualitative health research in the era of evidence-based practice. Qual. Health Res. 16 (10), 1371–1385.

Guba, E.G., 1990. The paradigm dialog. Sage Publications, Newbury Park.

Harding, J., 2006, "Grounded Theory," in The Sage Dictionary of Social Research Methods, V. Jupp, ed., Sage Publications, London, pp. 131–132.

Holloway, I. & Wheeler, S., 2010. Qualitative Research in Nursing and Healthcare, 3rd edn, Wiley-Blackwell, Chichester.

Hulscher, M.E.J.L., Wensing, M., van der Weijen, T., & Grol, R., 2006. Interventions to implement prevention in primary care. The Cochrane Database of Systematic Reviews no. 1. Art No: CD000362. pub2. DOI: 10. 1002/1465 1858. CD000362.pub2.

Jansen, Y.J.F.M., Foets, M.M.E., de Bont, A.A., 2009. The contribution of qualitative research to the development of tailor-made community–based interventions in primary care: a review. Eur. J. Public Health 20 (2), 220–226.

Johnson, R.B., Onwuegbuzie, A.J., Turner, L.A., 2007. Toward a Definition of Mixed Methods Research. Journal of Mixed Methods Research 1 (2), 112–133.

Keddie, V., 2006. "Case Study Method," in The Sage Book of Social Research Methods, V. Jupp, ed., Sage Publications, London, pp. 20–21.

Lempp, H., Kingsley, G., 2007. Qualitative assessments. Best practice & research. Clin. Rheumatol. 21 (5), 857–869.

Lewin, S., 2004. Mixing qualitative and quantitative methods in complex health service and public health RCTs: research 'best practice'. In: Mixed Methods in Health Services Research Conference, 23rd November 2004, Sheffield University.

Lincoln, Y.S., Guba, E.G., 1985. Naturalistic inquiry. Sage Publications, Newbury Park.

Mason, J., 2002. Qualitative Researching. 2nd Edition, Sage Publications Ltd London.

McEwan, M. J., Espie, C. A., & Metcalfe, J., 2004. "A systematic review of the contribution of qualitative research to the study of quality of life in children and adolescents with epilepsy", Seizure-European Journal of Epilepsy, vol. 13, no. 1, pp. 3–14.

Meadows-Oliver, M., 2009. Does qualitative research have a place in evidence-based nursing practice? J. Pediatr. Health Care 23 (5), 352–354.

Meyrick, J., 2006. What is good qualitative research? A first step towards a comprehensive approach to judging rigour/quality. J. Health Psychol. 11 (5), 799–808.

Nelson, A.M., 2008. Addressing the threat of evidence-based practice to qualitative inquiry through increasing attention to quality: A discussion paper. Int. J. Nurs. Stud. 45 (2), 316–322.

Newman, M., Thompson, C., Roberts, A.P., 2006. Helping practitioners understand the contribution of qualitative research to evidence-based practice. Evid. Based Nurs. 9 (1), 4–7.

Newton, J., 2006, "Action Research," in The Sage Dictionary of Social Research Methods, V. Jupp, ed., Sage Publications, London, pp. 2–3.

Ong, B. N. & Richardson, J. C., 2006. "The contribution of qualitative approaches to musculoskeletal research", Rheumatology vol. 45, no. 4, pp. 369–370.

Onwuegbuzie, A., Collins, K.M.T., 2007. A typology of mixed methods sampling designs in social science research. The Qualitative Report 12 (2), 281–316.

Petticrew, M., Roberts, H., 2003. Evidence, hierarchies, and typologies: horses for courses. J. Epidemiol. Community Health 57 (7), 527–529.

Pluye, P., Gagnon, M.P., Griffiths, F., Johnson-Lafleur, J., 2009. A scoring system for appraising mixed methods research, and concomitantly appraising qualitative, quantitative and mixed methods primary studies in Mixed Studies Reviews. Int. J. Nurs. Stud. 46 (4), 529–546.

Popay, J., Williams, G., 1998. Qualitative research and evidence-based healthcare. J. R. Soc. Med. 91 (35), 32–37.

Pope, C., Mays, N., 2006. Qualitative methods in health research. In: Pope, C., Mays, N. (Eds.), Qualitative Research in Health Care. Blackwell Publishing Ltd, Oxford, pp. 1–11.

Public Health Resource Unit England, 2006. Critical appraisal skills programme (CASP) Making sense of evidence. 10 questions to help you make sense of qualitative research. Public Health Resource Unit England, Oxford.

Rawlins, M., 2008. De testimonio: On the evidence for decisions about the use of therapeutic interventions. The Harveian Oration. Delivered before the Fellows of The Royal College of Physicians of London on Thursday 16 October 2008. The Royal College of Physicians, London.

Riessman, C. K., 1993. Narrative Analysis. Sage., Newbury Park, C. A.

Ritchie, J., Lewis, J., 2003. Qualitative research practice. A guide for social scientists. Sage Publications, London.

Rolfe, G., Gardner, L., 2006. Towards a geology of evidence-based practice–A discussion paper. Int. J. Nurs. Stud. 43 (7), 903–913.

Rycroft-Malone, J., Seers, K., Titchen, A., Harvey, G., Kitson, A., McCormack, B., 2004. What counts as evidence in evidence-based practice? J. Adv. Nurs. 47 (1), 81–90.

Sandelowski, M., 1998. Writing a good read: Strategies for re-presenting qualitative data. Res. Nurs. Health 21 (4), 375–382.

Sandelowski, M., Barroso, J., 2002. Reading Qualitative Studies. International Journal of Qualitative Methods 1 (1), 1.

Schumacher, K.L., Koresawa, S., West, C., Dodd, M., Paul, S.M., Tripathy, D., et al., 2005. Qualitative research contribution to a randomized clinical trial. Res. Nurs. Health 28 (3), 268–280.

Seale, C., 1999. The quality of qualitative research. Sage Publications Ltd, London.

Stake, R.E., 2010. Qualitative research. Studying how things work. Guildford Press, New York.

Stige, B., Malterud, K., Midtgarden, T., 2009. Toward an agenda for evaluation of qualitative research. Qual. Health Res. 19 (10), 1504–1516.

Strauss, A., Corbin, J., 1990. Basics of Qualitative Research. Grounded Theory Procedures and Techniques. Sage Ltd London.

van Manen, M., 1990. Researching lived experience, human science for an action sensitive pedagogy. State University of New York Press, New York.

Wolcott, H.F., 2002. Writing up qualitative research better. Qual. Health Res. 12 (1), 91–103.

Further reading

The National Centre for Social Research. A good resource for courses, publications and ideas. http://www.natcen.ac.uk/home.

Critical Appraisal Skills Programme. http://www.phru.nhs.uk/pages/phd/casp.htm.

Qualitative Research Guidelines Project. A useful website providing a comprehensive overview of some key evaluative (appraisal) criteria. http://www.qualres.org/index.html.

Qualitative Research Web Sites. Links to a range of websites covering all things qualitative. http://www.nova.edu/ssss/QR/web.html.

CHAPTER 5

Using evidence from quantitative studies

Gillian A Lancaster and Andrew C Titman

KEY POINTS

- The nature of quantitative inquiry.
- Hierarchy of evidence – identifying the appropriate research design for your clinical practice question.
- Understanding why critical appraisal is necessary.
- Assessing the quality of a study that asks a question about the effectiveness of a therapy or intervention.
- Assessing the quality of a study that asks a question about the accuracy of a particular diagnostic test or method of assessment.
- Assessing the quality of a study that asks a question about finding out the likely prognosis of a particular health problem or disease in relation to a defined set of risk factors.

- Developing a clinically useful interpretation of study results:
  - interpreting results from a study about the effectiveness of therapies: calculating odds ratios, risk ratios, relative risk reductions, absolute risk reductions and the number needed to treat
  - interpreting results from a study about the accuracy of a diagnostic test or assessment: calculating sensitivity, specificity, likelihood ratios, pre- and post-test odds
  - interpreting results from a study about prognosis or harm: calculating the number needed to harm.
  - using confidence intervals instead of 'p-values'.
- How to decide whether the results of a study can be applied to your patients and clinical setting.

Introduction

Quantitative research is a methodology based on experimentation and observation in which numerical information is collected using, for example, questionnaires or structured interviews, or is extracted from existing databases such as disease registers or other large surveys. Different research questions require evaluation through different study designs. Randomised controlled trials (RCTs) are the 'gold standard' study design for primary research upon which to base decisions on the effectiveness of healthcare interventions, but they are not appropriate, or ethical, for answering all questions. Observational study designs such as cohort studies, case-control studies and cross-sectional surveys define the nature of enquiry when we want to observe what is going on in the population of interest but we are not going to intervene in any way. A cohort study for example may be conducted prospectively and longitudinally, following and recording the progress of a cohort of participants over a number of years to see whether, in the light of their exposure history, they become diseased. On the other hand, for a case-control study we retrospectively go back in time to gather information on groups of diseased participants (cases) and non-diseased participants (controls) to compare whether or not having been exposed to certain risk factors for disease earlier in life (e.g. smoking history, exposure to sunburn as a child) has a bearing on getting the disease. Cross-sectional surveys observe a cross-section of people at some point or period in time to gain a 'snap-shot' of what is going on in the population in terms of the prevalence of certain diseases for example. Each design, therefore, has a slightly different strategy behind it.

There is no such thing as a perfect research study. Research is a real-world process and this means that researchers are often forced to compromise on certain aspects of the research and to modify the study design for lots of legitimate reasons. Similarly, it is important to realise that research is done on samples of a population who will never be identical to patients attending a community clinic or the patients in a ward. When designing a research study, researchers have to consider a number of key questions (Box 5.1). These questions apply in every type of research design. The decisions made by the researchers in response to these questions directly affect the degree to which the results of a study may be affected by bias. Bias refers to any influence or action in a study that distorts the findings (Burns & Grove 2001). In other words, any factor – for example, the way the sample is collected (selection bias) or the past length of time over which people are being asked to remember certain information (recall bias) – that leads to interventions appearing to be effective or risk factors for disease harmless when in fact

---

BOX 5.1 Questions to be considered in the design of a research study (adapted from Sim & Wright 2000)

What information (entities and variables) should be examined?
Under what conditions should this information be examined and collected?
What type(s) of data should be collected?
From whom should we collect these data?
At what time points (including follow-up) should data be collected?
What method should be employed for data collection?
How will the data be analysed?

they are not, or vice versa. The critical reader of research must always be aware that there may be multiple explanations for the findings reported in a study (Johnston 2005). Strategies for the minimisation of bias are now well known, and different strategies are required for different research designs and for the different stages of the study (Moore & McQuay 2000).

Hierarchy of evidence

Evidence that some research designs are more powerful than others has given rise to the notion of a hierarchy of evidence (Summerskill 2000). Figure 5.1 illustrates this hierarchy for studies relating to experimental designs that assess the effectiveness of therapies or interventions and for observational study designs that study known risk factors for disease. The higher a methodology appears on the continuum in the hierarchy, the more likely the results of such methods are to represent objective reality and hence the more certainty the practitioner has

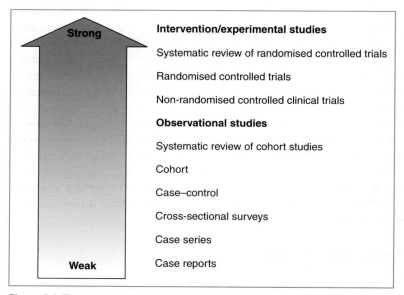

Figure 5.1 The hierarchy of evidence for questions about the effectiveness of an intervention/therapy or observed risk factors for disease

that the effect of interest will produce the associated health outcome (Johnston 2005). Such hierarchies provide a useful 'rule of thumb' against which to grade studies. Typologies of evidence are also used within the Government's National Service Frameworks and strategies (see http://www.nhs.uk/nhsengland/NSF/pages/Nationalserviceframeworks.aspx).

When looking for evidence about the effectiveness of interventions, well-conducted systematic reviews of RCTs or well-conducted RCTs provide the highest form of evidence. The process of randomisation means that the observed differences between the intervention group and the comparison group are more likely to be due to the intervention and not to other factors, such as patient, nurse or doctor preference (Matthews 2000). There will, however, always be circumstances where randomisation may be inappropriate or impossible, particularly in health service research (Bowling 1997). An obvious example is studies about harm or prognosis where it would not be ethical to give subjects a substance that was thought to be hazardous to their health.

The hierarchy of evidence shown in Figure 5.1 has led some clinicians to expressing concerns that the only questions considered to be important are those about effectiveness of interventions, and that the only valid type of study is the RCT (Evans & Pearson 2001, French 2002). In circumstances where there are clear reasons for not randomising, as we have seen already, observational studies have a vital role in providing evidence (Martin 2005). Furthermore, it would be inappropriate to conduct a RCT to answer a question such as 'How do young people with cancer, experience and manage fatigue?' Here the study aims to examine the experience of fatigue and explore influencing factors and management strategies adopted by young people with cancer, so a qualitative approach would be more appropriate.

Systematic reviews

In Figure 5.1, systematic reviews of RCTs feature at the top of the hierarchy of evidence about the effectiveness of interventions. A systematic review summarises pertinent research evidence on a defined health question, using explicit and rigorous methods (Cullinan 2005). In contrast to a traditional narrative review, which might simply reflect the findings of a few papers that support an author's particular point of view (Johnston 2005), a systematic review entails systematic and explicit methods for identifying, assessing and synthesising the available research evidence. This is an important distinction and highlights the biases associated with traditional, narrative reviews. There are numerous advantages to systematic reviews. For the busy practitioner, the most important advantage would seem to be their potential for aiding translation of research evidence into practice (Evans & Pearson 2001). A well-conducted review offers the clinician a rigorous distillation of the pertinent research evidence and recommendations for clinical practice and can help to overcome many of the practical and methodological limitations of individual studies (Chalmers & Altman 1995). Critical appraisal of systematic reviews is addressed separately in Chapter 6.

Why is critical appraisal necessary?

On a daily basis nurses and other health-care professionals are faced with a range of important clinical decisions. Practice based on evidence can decrease the uncertainty that patients and healthcare professionals experience in a complex and constantly evolving healthcare system. Not all published research evidence can be used for making decisions about patient care. Deficiencies in research design can make an intervention look better than it really is (Moher et al 1995). In addition, the location and participants of a particular research study may affect the results in a unique way. It is therefore necessary to assess the quality, interpretation of results and applicability of any research evidence that is being consulted to answer a specific clinical question. The process used to do this is known as critical appraisal and is a core skill for those wanting to use evidence in their practice.

Critical appraisal is a discipline for increasing the effectiveness of your reading, by encouraging systematic assessment of reports of research evidence to see which ones can best answer clinical problems and inform 'best practice' (O'Rourke 2005). The meaning of research evidence is most fully appreciated when considered within the context of clinical practice, where it can have a direct impact on clinical decisions. Clinical decisions are influenced not only by research evidence, but also by clinical expertise and patient preference (Sackett et al 1996). A variety of appraisal approaches can be used to determine the certainty and applicability of knowledge underpinning each of these three aspects of decision-making (Stevens 2005). In this chapter we focus on the appraisal of research evidence only and, specifically, quantitative research evidence. So, how do you critically appraise evidence produced through quantitative research designs? What does it demand of you?

Critical appraisal can be broken down into three distinct but related parts, as illustrated in Figure 5.2.

1. Are the results of the study valid? In other words, is the quality of the study good enough to produce results that can be used to inform clinical decisions?
2. What are the results and what do they mean for my patients?
3. Can I apply the results locally in my clinical setting?

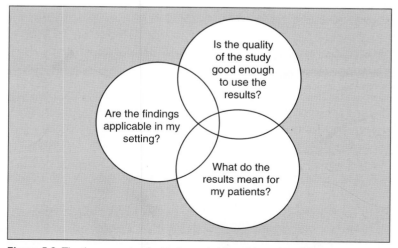

Figure 5.2 The three aspects of critical appraisal for evidence-based practice

Answering 'Yes' or 'No' to these questions can prove a challenge to healthcare practitioners. As Oxman et al (1993) observe, research evidence comes in shades of grey, rather than black and white: results *may* be valid, *might* show clinically important findings, *perhaps* will improve the patient's outcome.

Over the past 20 years or so, researchers and clinicians around the world have been working together to develop standard approaches to addressing these three questions. This work has led to the development of quality criteria for assessing the design of research studies. These criteria have been incorporated into critical appraisal checklists in the form of streamlined guides and toolkits that make the process of assessing studies much easier – see for example the 'Resource Centre' section of the Centre for Evidence Based Medicine website (www.cebm.net) and the NHS Solutions for Public Health website (http://www. sph.nhs.uk/what-we-do/public-health-workforce/resources/ critical-appraisals-skills-programme).

This chapter provides help in developing the skills and knowledge necessary to critically appraise quantitative studies. The chapter uses practical examples and exercises to illustrate the process: clinical scenarios are used to generate clinical questions and relevant published research papers are appraised (see website).

Are the results of the study valid?

One of the issues that all researchers face in the design and conduct of research in real-world settings is that of choosing a study design to minimise bias. When looked at from the perspective of research appraisers and consumers, strategies for minimising bias, referred to in the introduction, become quality criteria that can be used to assess the quality of a study. The strategies adopted by the researchers to minimise bias should be evident in the reporting of the research. Critical appraisal checklists are designed to summarise the bias minimisation strategies and help practitioners to ask the most relevant questions that will lead to a decision about the quality and usefulness of a paper.

Is the study design appropriate for the clinical question?

As shown in Chapter 2, the process of critical appraisal for evidence-based practice starts with the formulation of a question that arises from clinical practice. For critical appraisal purposes, clinical practice questions can, broadly speaking, be categorised into different types. In this chapter, we focus on clinical questions about:

- the effectiveness of a therapy or intervention
- the accuracy of a diagnostic test or other method of assessment
- the prognosis of a particular disease or health problem in relation to a given set of associated risk factors.

For each type of question there is a corresponding 'most appropriate' research design (overall plan or structure used by the researcher) that can be used to answer the question with a known degree of precision and minimal risk of bias (Blaikie 2000).

In this chapter we have focused on the optimal study design for three different types of questions, as illustrated in Table 5.1. However, it is important to remember that there may be good reasons why researchers choose to use study designs that at first appear to be less appropriate for the research question. Each research project presents unique challenges and a certain degree of flexibility is required by the researcher.

If the clinical question is about whether a particular intervention (e.g. a nurse-led discharge package) produces a certain outcome (e.g. decreased hospital stay), a study that compares length of hospital stay in a group receiving the intervention with length of stay in a group not receiving the intervention is required. There are a number of possible research designs that could be used for such a study but large, multicentred RCTs (or a systematic review of RCTs) are likely to give the best evidence of effectiveness (Gray 1997) provided they are conducted rigorously. In the case of questions about whether a particular diagnostic test or method of assessment performs well, a

TABLE 5.1 MATCHING STUDY DESIGN TO QUESTION

Type of question	Example question	Research design
The effectiveness of a therapy or intervention	Does the wearing of elastic compression stockings prevent deep vein thrombosis in long-haul flights?	Randomised controlled trial
The performance or accuracy of a particular diagnostic test/ method of assessment	In primary care, does asking patients about feeling depressed, experiencing loss of interest and needing help accurately identify those who are clinically depressed?	Study investigating test accuracy where a new method of assessment is compared with a reference standard test
Finding out the likely outcome of a particular health problem or disease in relation to a set of known risk factors (i.e. prognosis)	Are women oral contraceptive users who smoke at greater risk of myocardial infarction (MI)?	Cohort study: participants exposed to an agent (contraceptive pill) are followed forward in time to see if they develop an outcome (MI)

Case-control study: participants with the condition (MI) are matched with controls (no MI). Study looks back in time to identify exposure to an agent (contraceptive pill) |

study design that compares the accuracy of a new test when used on people with and without the target condition against a reference standard will be most appropriate (Mant 1999a). We will refer to this design as a diagnostic test study. Where the question is about the most likely outcome of a particular health problem (i.e. the prognosis) in the light of a number of associated risk factors, the most appropriate design will be one that measures relevant outcomes in individuals with (exposed to) and without (not exposed to) the relevant risk factor over a sufficient period of time (Mant 1999b). As we have already seen the two appropriate study designs for this type of question are the cohort study and the case-control study. In our exercises we will be using a set of tools developed by the Critical Appraisal Skills Programme (CASP 2010) that have been created specifically to appraise these four different types of study design: namely (i) a randomised controlled trial (CASP 2006a), (ii) a diagnostic test study (CASP 2006b), (iii) a cohort study (CASP 2004) and (iv) a case-control study (CASP 2006c).

Regardless of the type of study, a rigorous approach to the design, conduct, analysis and reporting stages of the study is important in view of the effect that each of these stages can have on the results. For example, RCTs with methodological shortfalls, such as failure to conceal from the patient and assessor the group to which the patient has been allocated, tend to overestimate treatment effects (Matthews 2000). Similarly diagnostic test studies that only choose a sample of confirmed diseased and non-diseased people and exclude the broad spectrum of people in between (e.g. with early mild or moderate symptoms), tend to inflate estimates of test performance (Lijmer et al 1999).

General points to consider when assessing quality criteria for the three types of clinical question that we are considering are given below. These points should be considered when attempting the exercises found on the website.

Points to consider when assessing the quality of a study that asks a question about the effectiveness of a therapy or intervention

- The importance of randomisation has already been discussed: it is a powerful technique where the aim is to ensure that, as far as possible, the two groups are similar in every respect apart from the fact that one group is given the intervention. This then means that any difference in outcome between the two groups is likely to be due to the intervention. A computer-generated random number sequence is one example of an appropriate randomisation method. An approach that allocates people to the two groups for example by treating on alternate days is a weaker method of allocation, but may sometimes be the only feasible method.

- The group to which the patient has been allocated must be concealed from the clinician/researcher until the patient has (at least) been accepted into the trial. This is referred to as allocation concealment and is an important factor in reducing bias. If the clinician believes that the patient may benefit from the treatment, and realises that the patient is due to be allocated to the control group, he or she may consciously or subconsciously dissuade the patient from participating in the trial. Ideally, randomisation should be carried out by someone removed from the project using, for example, sequentially numbered sealed, opaque envelopes. Allocation based on criteria such as date of birth or alternate days are not recommended as clinicians will be able to work out the next allocation sequence.

- Where possible, patients, clinicians and researchers should continue to be 'blinded' as to whether a patient is in the treatment or control group. If patients know that they are in the control group, they may feel that they have received substandard care and may, as a result, alter their behaviour. Similarly, clinicians may consciously or subconsciously take compensatory measures for patients who are in the control group (for example, by offering alternative therapies or additional support). Any difference in the treatment effects between the two groups may be due to this additional attention rather than the intervention. The researcher may have preconceived ideas about the treatment and, where the outcomes of interest are fairly subjective, these preconceptions may influence the way in which the researcher interprets and analyses the data. Clearly, blinding is not possible in all studies but attempts should be made to blind one (single-blind) or all (double-blind/treble-blind) of the above groups of people.

- People drop out of studies for all sorts of reasons: death, move away from the area, treatment too unpleasant, etc. It is important that the researcher tries to identify whether the reasons relate to the outcomes of interest or not as this may have a bearing on the analysis. The analysis should ideally be done on an 'intention to treat' basis: patients are analysed in the groups to which they were randomised regardless of whether they swap from the intervention arm of the trial to the control arm or vice versa. If participants in the treatment group stop taking a drug because they feel worse (and blame the drug), and are then included in the control group, the drug may appear to be more effective than it really is due to exclusion of those patients with poor outcomes from the treatment group.

- Sample size is another important consideration – did the researchers explicitly estimate how many people were needed in order to detect the minimum clinically worthwhile difference that they want to detect between groups? Studying more people than is necessary wastes resources, whilst studying too few people might lead to results that reflect chance variation rather than the real situation. To illustrate, in a trial of 10 participants, where five are randomised to receive drug A and five to receive drug B, and where the outcomes are the same for both groups, this could mean one of two things: either there is no difference between the drugs or one of the drugs is more effective, but because of the small sample this difference is not detected (Kirkwood 1988). A 'power calculation' will provide an estimation of the required sample size. The power of a study is the probability of detecting a significant result if the difference between outcomes in the two groups is really there.

- The comparison of demographic and health status details for the two randomised groups is good practice at the start of the study. Apparent differences between the two groups, for example differences in age, co-morbid conditions, gender or disease severity, could potentially affect the results of the study. The groups should ideally be similar for any variables that are likely to influence outcome. Similarity between groups is not always achieved by randomisation, even where the methods of randomisation are adequate.

- It is helpful if the intervention is described in sufficient detail to allow clinicians to reproduce it in their own setting. In addition, the primary outcome in which the investigators would expect to see a clinically important difference should be given, along with details of how the outcome was to be measured. Measurement instruments which have been validated outside the study and found to measure what they purport to measure, and which are sensitive, appropriate and acceptable, inspire more confidence than measurement instruments that have not been validated. Similarly they should be consistently reliable when used on different occasions or by different assessors.

Points to consider when assessing the quality of a study that asks a question about the performance or accuracy of a particular diagnostic test

- The 'new' test should be compared against the method that is currently regarded as 'the best' (i.e. the reference standard) and it is important that both tests should be applied in all participants. It is also important that the reference standard correctly diagnoses participants since the 'new' test is being compared in terms of its accuracy to this 'gold' standard.

- An appropriate spectrum of patients (i.e. patients with mild, moderate and severe forms of the condition) should ideally be included in the study, with details of the proportions in each of these groups reported. A test may be able to identify people who are severely ill, but not those with a mild form of the condition.

- Ideally, a consecutive sample of participants who fulfil the inclusion criteria should be tested, or alternatively a random sample selected from a register if such a list of participants was available. This ensures that individuals are not inappropriately 'selected out' of the study, thereby affecting the results and conclusions of the study. The participants should be representative of the type of participants to which the test will be administered in practice and should be taken from the appropriate setting.

- It is recommended that the clinician or investigator is 'blinded' to the results of the test that is carried out first. If the clinician suspects from the initial test that the patient does not have the disease in question, he or she may decide to avoid subjecting the patient to the second test. Blinding also avoids the conscious and unconscious bias of causing the reference standard to be overinterpreted when the diagnostic test is positive and underinterpreted when it is negative (Sackett et al 2000).

- Reliability (reproducibility) of a test needs to be considered: the results of tests carried out by different individuals or by the same individual at different times should remain unchanged, provided the true underlying variable being measured remains the same. Disagreement between two examiners is called interobserver variability, and disagreement within one examiner over time is called intraobserver variability. In tests that are not reproducible, it is difficult to know whether a true measurement is being obtained. This creates problems in research and in clinical practice.

Points to consider when assessing the quality of a study that asks a question about the likely prognosis or outcome of a particular health problem or disease in relation to a set of risk factors

- It is important that the participants in the study are truly 'at risk' of getting the disorder or truly have the disorder of interest (depending upon the design), and that they are entering the study at a common point in the course of their disease. In a cohort study aiming to identify the risk of renal disease in people with diabetes, for example, if some of the participants already have undiagnosed mild kidney damage at the start of the study, this could influence the results in a negative way. Entry or eligibility criteria are, therefore, required and should be clearly specified.

- Length of observation (or follow-up) should be adequate for all possible outcomes (especially negative outcomes). If participants, for example people who have smoked 20 or more cigarettes a day for 1 year, are followed up for 4 years to establish risk of lung cancer, the conclusions of the study are likely to be very different than if followed up for 15 years.

- People are inevitably lost to follow-up during the course of a cohort study and the reasons for this should be explored and closely monitored. If participants are lost to follow-up through death rather than because they feel better, and this information is known to the researcher, he or she can take this into consideration when presenting the results.

- Measurement of outcomes and exposures can be a source of bias, especially where the measure is subjective (e.g. quality of life) or sensitive (e.g. sexual abuse in childhood), or where a number of different assessors have taken measurements over the course of the study. The method of measurement should, therefore, be clearly defined in advance and regular training given as necessary. In addition, where measurement requires a degree of judgement, the person taking the measurement or doing the assessment should remain blind to the patient's condition.

- When observing health outcomes, it is important to take account of the factors or variables that can affect health. In longitudinal studies, time itself acts as a confounding variable. As people get older they develop more illness regardless of any other factors. The effect of such confounding variables can be taken into account in the process of data analysis.

For a more detailed discussion of each set of points, readers are referred to the *Users' Guides to the Medical Literature manual* of the American Medical Association (Guyatt et al 2008) or the related 'Users' guides to the medical literature' series published in JAMA (Laupacis et al 1994).

To illustrate assessment of the quality of a research study, we use the clinical scenario given in Box 5.2, which is concerned with whether the occurrence of deep-vein thrombosis when flying can be reduced by wearing elastic stockings. A search for evidence on the topic has revealed a paper by Scurr et al (2001). Table 5.2 shows a worked example using criteria to assess the quality of the study that is asking a question about the effectiveness of an intervention.

BOX 5.2 Example of a study assessing the effectiveness of an intervention

Scenario: Mrs Pink is taking her son Henry and her parents to Disney World in Florida, and they have booked a long-haul flight. Mum is worried about her parents, although both are fit and well, after reading an article in a women's magazine about the risk of deep vein thrombosis (DVT) and the benefits of wearing elastic stockings during the flight. She asks for your help in deciding what to do. You search for information on the web and find a relevant paper in the Lancet.

Clinical question: Do compression stockings prevent DVT in the lower limbs during long-haul air travel?

Evidence: Scurr J H, Machin S J, Bailey-King S, Mackie I J, McDonald S, Coleridge Smith P D 2001 Frequency and prevention of symptomless deep-vein thrombosis in long-haul flights: a randomized trial. Lancet 357:1485–1489.

Results reported in the study: The results for DVT and superficial thrombophlebitis (SVT), assessed within 48 hours of the passengers' return flight, are presented. For those passengers allocated to the stocking group, 0 out of 115 had DVT compared to 12 out of 116 passengers not wearing compression stockings. With regard to SVT, 4 out of 115 passengers wearing stockings developed SVT compared to 0 out of 116 in the no-stocking group.

TABLE 5.2 ASSESSING THE QUALITY OF A STUDY THAT INVESTIGATES WHETHER A PARTICULAR INTERVENTION IS EFFECTIVE: A WORKED EXAMPLE USING THE CASP CHECKLIST 'TEN QUESTIONS TO HELP YOU MAKE SENSE OF RANDOMISED CONTROLLED TRIALS' (CASP 2006a, WITH PERMISSION)

Type of question	Assessment criteria	Response (Yes/Can't tell/No)	Comment
Screening question	Did the study ask a clearly focused question?	Yes	This study sought to determine the frequency of deep vein thrombosis (DVT) in the lower limb in middle-aged men and women during long-haul economy class air travel and the efficacy of elastic compression stockings in its prevention.
	Was this a randomised controlled trial (RCT), and was it appropriately so?	Yes	This study compared the frequency and prevention of DVT in two groups randomly allocated to wear or not wear stockings. The study design (RCT) is appropriate for investigating the effectiveness of an intervention.
Detailed questions	Were participants appropriately allocated to intervention and control groups?	Yes	The author states that passengers were randomly allocated to receive compression stocking (n=115) or no stockings (n=116); however, the method of randomisation is not described. Sealed envelopes were used to conceal from the investigators and passengers which group the passengers were to be allocated to.

(Continued)

TABLE 5.2 (CONTINUED)

Type of question	Assessment criteria	Response (Yes/ Can't tell/No)	Comment
	Were participants, staff and study personnel 'blind' to participants' study group?	Can't tell	Not possible to blind the passengers or the staff administering the stockings. They all knew who was receiving treatment. It might have been possible to blind the laboratory staff and the ultrasonographer, but there is a high risk that the patients might have revealed to the ultrasonographer which group they were in.
	Were all the participants who entered the trial accounted for at its conclusion?	Yes	Yes, trial profile clearly describes and states intention to treat in the analysis section. Data on all participants originally randomised have been included in the analysis.
			The authors show the numbers of passengers lost to follow-up for each group. These appear to be equally distributed between groups.
	Were the participants in all groups followed up and data collected in the same way?	Can't tell	This is unclear; insufficient information is provided about the actual study procedure. It would be difficult to comment on the influence of performance bias.

Did the study have enough participants to minimise the play of chance?	Can't tell	This was described as a pilot study and, therefore, no power calculation was undertaken.
How are the results presented and what is the main result?		Presented as a proportion of participants experiencing DVT after airline travel. None of the participants wearing stockings had a DVT. Although an increased risk of superficial thrombophlebitis in varicose veins if the stockings are worn is reported, the increase is not statistically significant. Ten per cent (n=12/116) of participants not wearing stockings developed a symptomless DVT. The authors conclude that wearing an elasticated stocking during long-haul air travel is associated with a reduction in symptomless DVT.
How precise are the results?		Confidence intervals are reported for each group, not between groups, but are indicative of clinical significance.
Were all the important outcomes considered so the results can be applied?	No	A number of limitations were addressed in the paper that would need to be considered such as in-flight behaviours, e.g. walking, and drinking water, and the effect these may have had on the results. The reported risk of thrombophlebitis in varicose veins if the stockings are worn would also need to be taken into consideration.

What do the results of the study mean for my patients?

Once you have decided the quality of the study is good enough and the results can be applied in your setting, the next stage is to interpret what the results of the study mean for your individual patients. This is the second aspect of critical appraisal (Fig. 5.2). It is a common misperception that evidence-based practice is all about statistics. We hope that it is already clear that this is not the case. The evidence-based practice approach is that the statistical analyses carried out in a study are not the most important consideration when critically appraising a paper. Most important is the choice and quality of the study design. If a study was well designed for the research question being asked, then there is a high probability that the researchers' interpretation of the results can be trusted (Sackett et al 2000). Even well-done statistical analysis cannot compensate for bias caused by deficiencies in the study design. When critically appraising a research study, the reader does not have to be an expert in statistics. However, it is useful if the reader is able to calculate and interpret different effect measures, taking into account both the statistical significance and clinical importance of the results.

Effect measures

A number of clinically meaningful effect measures have been developed for different types of clinical questions and study designs. These include measures such as the odds ratio (OR), relative risk/risks ratio (RR), relative risk reduction (RRR) and absolute risk reduction (ARR). One increasingly popular measure is the number needed to treat (NNT), which is useful for interpreting results from studies about the effectiveness of a therapy or intervention (Laupacis et al 1988). NNT shows how many patients have to be given the intervention for one extra person to benefit who would not have done so if given the comparison treatment. A similar measure is the number needed to harm (NNH) which is used for interpreting the results of prognostic/harm studies. Studies looking at a particular method of diagnosis or assessment often give the results of the test in terms of its sensitivity (proportion of people with a condition who test positively when using the new test) and specificity (proportion of people without the condition who test negatively when using the new test). These results can be converted (using likelihood ratios) into probabilities that express how likely the diagnosis is for a particular patient.

More studies are being published that use these types of measures to report their results, but healthcare practitioners still need to understand how to calculate these themselves. At first some of the calculations may seem a bit intimidating. However, despite their apparent complexity, they usually only involve some simple arithmetic that can, if necessary, be done with pencil and paper. The most effective way of learning these techniques is by working through real examples. The following sections will describe how these measures are calculated and interpreted, along with associated confidence intervals, using as examples results taken from the papers summarized in Boxes 5.2 (used in the worked example above), 5.3 and 5.4.

BOX 5.3 Example of a study assessing the performance of a diagnostic assessment tool

Scenario: Thomas Davies, a 45-year-old frequent attender at his local GP surgery, visits the practice nurse. He has been unemployed for 6 months, has no mental health problems, but self-reports that he is 'feeling down and has a loss of interest'. He hardly ever attended the surgery until 3 months ago. Nurse feels that he has a 50% chance of having clinical depression (which means he has a 50% chance of not having clinical depression) but she wants to be more certain before referring him for a specialist assessment. She knows you have recently been on a critical appraisal course and asks you to help her find some more information before deciding what to do. You search on the web and find a paper in the BMJ which might be useful.

Clinical question: In patients with clinical depression, how accurately does patient response to three simple questions (two screening questions and a question relating to help) diagnose clinical depression?

Evidence: Arroll B, Goodyear-Smith F, Kerse N, Fishman T, Gunn J 2005 Effect of the addition of a 'help' question to two screening questions on specificity for diagnosis of depression in general practice: diagnostic validity study. British Medical Journal 331: 884–889

Results reported in the study: A positive response to 'either screening question and the help question' had a sensitivity of 96% (95% CI 86–99%) and a specificity of 89% (95% CI 87–91%).

BOX 5.4 Example of a study on prognosis assessing the association between a surgical outcome and exposure to risk factors

Scenario: Lydia Pierce is a 7-year-old girl who is due to have a tonsillectomy due to chronic tonsillitis. Lydia suffers from asthma and her mother, Jane, is a heavy smoker. As Jane's friend you are worried that there may be complications to the surgery due to Lydia's respiratory problems and the fact that she has been exposed to passive smoking all her life. You find a relevant journal article of a recent study carried out at a children's hospital in Perth, Australia.

Clinical question: Are children with a past history of respiratory problems including passive smoke exposure, at a higher risk of adverse respiratory events during or soon after surgical intervention?

Evidence: Von Ungern-Sternberg BS, Boda K, Chambers NA, Rebmann C, Johnson C, Sly PD, Habre W 2010 Risk assessment for respiratory complications in paediatric anaesthesia: a prospective cohort study. Lancet 376:773–783.

Results reported in the study: Children who have a previous history of respiratory problems (e.g. a recent upper respiratory tract infection, asthma and wheezing during the past 12 months, passive smoke exposure) have a threefold increase in the risk of peri-operative respiratory adverse events; that is, 31% of children with a history of respiratory problems compared to 10% of children without a history of respiratory problems.

Calculating effect measures for testing a therapy or intervention

A 2 × 2 table like the one shown in Figure 5.3 is a standard tool for calculating clinically meaningful results. Each cell in the table contains a number and is labelled with a letter – a, b, c and d. In a comparative study participants are divided into two groups: the group that received the 'new' or experimental therapy (cells a and b) and the group that did not (cells c and d). The presence (cells a and c) or absence (cells b and d) of the outcome of interest is reported for both groups. The letters in the cells are used in the formulae for calculating summary measures

		Outcome: Deep vein thrombosis		Totals	
		Present	Absent		
Study groups	Experimental group (compression stockings)	a 0	b 115	a + b 115	
	Control group (no compression stockings)	c 12	d 104	c + d 116	
Totals		a + c 12	b + d 219	a + b + c + d 231	

Figure 5.3 A 2 × 2 table for interpreting results of a study on the effectiveness of an intervention with data from the study by Scurr and colleagues (2001) described in Box 5.2

like the OR, RR, RRR, ARR and NNT (Table 5.3). The numbers to go in each cell are obtained from the study results. It is often possible to calculate the numbers if they are not given. Figure 5.3 uses the results from the study conducted by Scurr and colleagues (2001) summarised in Box 5.2.

The formulae for calculating different effect measures are given in Table 5.3. In this section we will focus specifically on the ARR and the NNT, an increasingly popular way of presenting the results of controlled clinical trials. In a trial comparing an experimental treatment with a control treatment, the NNT is the estimated number of patients who need to be treated with the experimental treatment for one additional patient to benefit (Altman 1998). The smaller the NNT, the more important the treatment effect. In the example (Box 5.2) the ARR is 10%, indicating that the absolute benefit of stockings is a 10% reduction in the rate of DVT. The NNT is 10 (the figure is typically rounded up toward the more conservative whole number). This means that 10 long-haul flight passengers need to wear compression stockings to prevent one extra passenger from developing symptomless DVT. When presenting any measure of effect, the 95% confidence intervals should also be presented. Box 5.5 demonstrates how the confidence intervals can be calculated

TABLE 5.3 CALCULATING EFFECTS MEASURES

Measure	Description	Formula	Example
Odds ratio (OR)	The odds of an event (outcome) in the experimental group divided by the odds of an event in the control group. Usually expressed as a decimal number. An OR of 1 indicates no difference between the two groups (value of 'no effect')	$(a/b)/(c/d) = ad/bc$	$(0/115)/(12/104)$ $= (0 \times 104)/(115 \times 12)$ $= 0$
Risk ratio (RR) Also known as relative risk or rate ratio	The risk of an event in the experimental group (known as the experimental event rate (EER)) divided by the risk of an event in the control group (known as the control event rate (CER)). Usually expressed as a decimal number. A RR of 1 indicates no difference between the two groups	$(a/(a+b))/(c/(c+d))$	$(0/115)/(12/116)$ $= 0/0.1$ $= 0$

Absolute risk reduction (ARR) Also known as risk difference or rate difference	The risk of an event in the control group (the control event rate (CER)) minus the risk of an event in the experimental group (the experimental event rate (EER)). Usually expressed as a percentage. An ARR of 0% indicates no difference between the two groups	$c/(c + d) - a/(a + b)$ $(12/116) - (0/(115)$ $= 0.1 - 0$ $= 0.1 (10\%)$
Relative risk reduction (RRR)	The ARR divided by the risk of an event in the control group. Can also be calculated as $1 - RR$. Usually expressed as a percentage. A RRR of 0 indicates no difference between the two groups	$ARR/(c/(c + d))$ also $1 - RR$ $0.1/(12/116)$ or $1 - 0 = 1 (100\%)$
Number needed to treat (NNT)	The reciprocal of the ARR. Usually expressed as a whole number	$NNT = 1/ARR$ $1/0.1 = 10$

BOX 5.5 Calculating 95% confidence intervals for the ARR and NNT

Formula 95% CI for ARR:

$$= ARR \pm 1.96 \sqrt{\frac{EER(100 - EER)}{a+b} + \frac{CER(100 - CER)}{c+d}}$$

Example using data from the study by Scurr et al 2001:

$$95\% \text{ CI for ARR} = 10 \pm 1.96 \sqrt{\frac{0(100-0)}{115} + \frac{10(100-10)}{116}}$$

95% CI for ARR = 10 ± 5.5%
Formula 95% CI for NNT = 100/upper 95% CI to 100/lower 95% CI of the ARR

Example using data from the study by Scurr et al 2001
95% CI for NNT = 100/15.5 to 100/4.5
95% CI for NNT = 6 to 22

for both the ARR and NNT. For the ARR the 95% confidence interval is 4.5% to 15.5%, indicating that we are 95% certain that the true absolute benefit may be as low as 4.5% or as high as 15.5%. Given that the confidence intervals do not include the value of 'no effect', we can see that the results are statistically significant. The 95% confidence interval for NNT is 6 to 22. The results suggest that wearing elastic stockings during the flight does seem beneficial.

Calculating effect measures for assessing the performance or accuracy of a diagnostic test

In a study that tests whether a diagnostic test or assessment works, the new test is compared to an existing 'gold standard', which it is assumed diagnoses the target condition with certainty. In the study given in the example in Box 5.3 (Arroll et al 2005) the gold standard is the score obtained using the Composite International Diagnostic Interview (CIDI). All patients (with and without the condition) receive both the new test and the

		Outcome: Depression as diagnosed by CIDI		Totals
		Present	Absent	
New test: 'two screening questions plus help question'	Positive	a 45	b 94	a + b 139
	Negative	c 2	d 795	c + d 797
Totals		a + c 47	b + d 889	a + b + c + d 936*

* 1025 patients agreed to participate; 936 completed the CIDI.

Figure 5.4 A 2 × 2 table for interpreting results of a study on the accuracy of a diagnostic assessment with data from the study by Arroll and colleagues (2005) described in Box 5.3

gold standard test. Figure 5.4 shows a 2 × 2 table complete with data from the study. The results of diagnostic studies are usually reported in terms of sensitivity (in our example, this would be the probability of having a positive result using 'either screening question plus help question' if you have depression) and specificity (the probability of having a negative result using 'either screening question plus help question' if you do not have depression). A high sensitivity is a useful result because the presence of a negative test result in a patient virtually rules out a positive diagnosis. In this example (sensitivity 96%), we could say that if Mr Davies answers 'no' to the screening questions plus help question, we can be fairly sure that he does not have depression (we would only be wrong in four patients out of 100). A high specificity is a useful result because a positive test result in an individual patient effectively rules in a positive diagnosis. In this example (specificity 89%), if Mr Davies answers 'yes' to either screening question plus the help question, we could be reasonably sure that he had clinical depression. Eleven patients in 100 answer 'yes' to one of the questions but do not have clinical depression. The 95% confidence intervals for sensitivity and specificity given in Box 5.3 suggest that the estimates are fairly precise, with both lower limits remaining above 85%. Whilst the sensitivity and specificity are useful when they are high, it is rare for both the sensitivity and specificity to be high on the same test as there is nearly always a trade-off between the two.

In addition, the performance of a test is affected by the prevalence of the condition in the underlying population. In an individual patient, this is referred to as the pre-test probability of an individual having the condition. In our scenario the nurse thought that Mr Davies had a pre-test probability of 50% of having clinical depression. What the nurse wants the test to do is to either increase or decrease this probability to indicate more strongly whether he does or does not have depression respectively. This is called the post-test probability.

In practice what we need to know is, does testing 'positive' or 'negative' help us to determine whether the patient does or does not have the disease of interest? Technically we can think of this as the likelihood that a positive test result is a true positive and that a negative test result is a true negative. The ratio of true-positive results to false-positive results is known as the positive likelihood ratio. The ratio of true-negative results to false-negative results is known as the negative likelihood ratio. We can calculate these from the sensitivity and specificity respectively. The formulae for calculating these measures are given in Table 5.4.

The interpretation of likelihood ratios depends partly on the underlying prevalence (Mant 1999c). If we convert the prevalence into pre-test odds, and multiply the pre-test odds by the negative or positive likelihood ratio, then we can calculate the post-test odds. Most people are more comfortable with using probability than odds, so we can then convert the post-test odds back into a post-test probability of disease. In our scenario the nurse thought that Mr Davies had a pre-test probability of 50% of having clinical depression (and a 50% probability of not having clinical depression). The pre-test probability of 50:50, which is the same as pre-test odds of 1:1, can be combined with the likelihood ratio to give us the post-test odds or probability. In this example 1:1 can be multiplied with the likelihood ratio 8.7, giving post-test

TABLE 5.4 FORMULAE FOR CALCULATING USEFUL CLINICAL MEASURES FOR ANSWERING QUESTIONS ABOUT WHETHER A PARTICULAR DIAGNOSTIC TEST OR METHOD OF ASSESSMENT WORKS

Measure	Formula	Example
Sensitivity	a/a + c	45/47 = 0.96 or 96%
Specificity	d/b + d	795/889 = 0.89 or 89%
Positive likelihood ratio	Sensitivity/(100 − specificity)	96/(100 − 89) = 8.7
Negative likelihood ratio	(100 - sensitivity)/ specificity	(100 − 96)/89 = 0.04
Pre-test odds	Prevalence/100 - prevalence	50/(100 − 50) = 1
Post-test odds	Pre-test odds × likelihood ratio	1 × 8.7 = 8.7
Post-test probability	Post-test odds/(post-test odds + 1)	8.7/(8.7 + 1) = 89.7%

odds of 8.7:1 in favour of clinical depression. If you are more comfortable with probability than odds, post-test odds of 8.7:1 converts to a more useful, but not diagnostic, post-test probability of 89.7%. This increase in the probability of depression following the test suggests that Mr Davies may well be clinically depressed and a more detailed assessment by a psychologist may be helpful to firmly establish the correct diagnosis.

Note that a simple way of summarising post-test probabilities for a range of pre-test probabilities and likelihood ratios is by using a special diagram called a nomogram (see Sackett et al 2000 for further information).

Calculating effect measures for prognostic studies

Studies of prognosis/harm usually report results in terms of proportions or rates of events in the two groups being compared. If we are satisfied that the evidence from a study is of good enough quality to use, then we need to decide if the association between exposure and outcome is sufficiently strong and convincing for us to have to do something about it. For the scenario given in Box 5.4 related to the paper by von Ungern-Sternberg et al (2010) the result of interest is the difference between the rate of peri-operative respiratory adverse events in children who had a previous history of respiratory problems compared to those who had no previous history of respiratory problems. A 2 × 2 table can be used to aid interpretation of the study results and is given in Figure 5.5.

The researchers did quite appropriately adjust the results for other potential confounding variables such as age, but these results are not shown in the paper. In this example the absolute risk difference between the two groups is 21%, as shown in Table 5.5, with 95% confidence interval 19 to 23%. In general, the research question of the study will determine the importance of the size of the effect measure. For example, if the outcome is mortality, a difference of 1% may be considered sufficient to change practice. If the outcome is benefit obtained by using a very expensive drug with unpleasant side effects, a difference of 1% may not be considered sufficient to change practice. Here, the adverse events are rarely fatal so we may be willing to accept a higher absolute risk difference than we would if the outcome was mortality.

| | | Outcome: Peri-operative adverse respiratory event | | Totals |
		Yes	No	
History of respiratory problems	Yes	a 699	b 1557	a + b 2256
	No	c 693	d 6348	c + d 7041
Totals		a + c 1392	b + d 7905	a + b + c + d 9297

Figure 5.5 A 2 × 2 table for interpreting results of a study on prognosis/harm with data from the study by von Ungern-Sternberg and colleagues (2010) described in Box 5.4

TABLE 5.5 FORMULAE FOR CALCULATING USEFUL CLINICAL MEASURES
FOR ANSWERING QUESTIONS ABOUT PROGNOSIS/HARM

Measure	Formula	Example
Relative risk (RR)	(a/(a + b))/ (c/(c + d))	(699/2256)/(693/7041) = 3.15
Absolute risk	(a/(a + b)) − (c/(c + d))	(699/2256)−(693/7041) = 0.211
Number needed to harm (NNH)	1/ARI	1/0.211 = 4.7

Another result reported in the study is RR (Table 5.5). This measures the relative difference in the percentage affected by respiratory adverse events in each group. In this example the RR tells us that the risk of peri-operative respiratory problems is 3.1 times greater amongst children with a previous history of respiratory problems compared to those with no previous history. As a general rule of thumb, in cohort studies we can say that an RR increase of more than 3 is unlikely to be the result of bias (Sackett et al 2000). From the results of the paper we can deduce that there is a difference in risk between the two groups and that this difference is unlikely to be the result of bias. But is the difference large enough to recommend a change of anaesthetic management for Lydia?

To fully assess the clinical relevance of the findings we can calculate an additional measure. Table 5.5 shows the formula for calculating the number needed to harm (NNH), for which we first need to calculate the absolute risk increase (ARI). The ARI tells us the size of the difference between the two groups which is 21% (or 0.211 from Table 5.5). The ARI in this example tells us that the difference between the groups is equivalent to 211 events per 1000 children. The NNH tells us the number of operations involving children with a history of respiratory problems that would have to take place for one extra adverse respiratory event. In the example, the NNH = 5, i.e. not many operations at all. In this case, we can conclude that Lydia's respiratory problems do put her at increased risk of suffering an adverse event during or shortly after her operation. However, since she has had neither an upper respiratory tract infection recently nor any wheezing with exercise, then it should be safe for Lydia to go ahead and have her tonsillectomy.

p-values and confidence intervals

The way the results of research are reported can often make it difficult to apply them in daily clinical practice. One reason for this is that one of the major concerns of researchers is to establish the likelihood of their result being caused by chance variation. The p-value is frequently presented to illustrate this likelihood. Its value always lies between zero and one. A p-value of 0.5 would tell us that there is a 1 in 2 (50%) probability of observing our data (or data even more extreme) if there is no real effect (i.e. if the null hypothesis is true). If this were the case, we would be unlikely to accept the results of the study as being significant. Conventionally, we accept a p-value of 0.05 or below as being statistically significant. That means that a significant result could occur 5 times out of 100 (or 1 time in 20) when, in fact, there is really no difference between the groups being compared. Some papers may use a more rigorous cut-off point of p equal to 0.01 or below as statistically significant (a 1 in 100 probability). The p-value alone does not give any indication of the size or direction of the difference (or treatment effect) (Gardner & Altman 1986). Therefore, it does not help you assess what the likely effect will be on your patient.

Health-related research studies may present results accompanied by confidence intervals, which provide more information than the p-value alone. A formal definition of a confidence interval is 'a range of values for a variable of interest constructed so that this range has a specified probability of including the true value of the variable' (Last 1988). The accepted convention is to use the 95% confidence interval. This means that you can be 95% certain that the true value of the variable of interest lies within the upper and lower limits of the confidence interval.

Confidence intervals are a clinically useful way of measuring the precision of an estimate of effect size. When evaluating the effect of an intervention, a confidence interval not only provides us with information on statistical significance, but also indicates with a certain degree of confidence (e.g. 95% or 95 times out of 100) the range within which the true treatment effect is likely to lie. If, when comparing interventions, the confidence interval includes the value of 'no effect', then the difference between the two intervention groups is not statistically significant. The narrower the gap between the upper and lower 95% confidence interval limits, the more certain we will be about the precision of the estimate. The 95% confidence interval can be calculated for most common statistical estimates.

Can I apply the results in my clinical setting?

So far we have dealt with the quality of health-related research studies – how well has a study been conducted for the research question being asked, and how to calculate and interpret the results. But can we trust the study's results enough to apply them in our own clinical setting? What needs to be recognised here is that not all high-quality studies are applicable to all patients or all clinical settings. Health-related research takes place all over the world, in settings that may be very different from the one in which your patients are found. In addition, there is a tendency for studies to include 'scientifically clean' populations (Greenhalgh 1997), excluding patients who have co-existing illnesses or additional risk factors. This can mean that patients included in health-related research are often very different from those seen in everyday clinical practice. The context in which you practise and/ or the context in which each patient's consultation takes place is, to some degree, unique. Alongside the assessment of a study's quality, it is important to consider whether the results obtained can be applied to your patient's and your clinical setting. Can the results of a trial recruiting patients aged 18–50 years be applied to patients over 60 years of age? If a study has been conducted in Brazil, what do the results mean with regard to patients being treated in the UK?

It is unlikely that the patients and settings used in a research study will ever be identical to yours. When addressing the issue of applicability, we need to consider the extent to which differences in patients and settings might affect the results. Are the differences so great that we might expect the direction of effect to alter? If the differences would only change the size or extent of the effect of the treatment, rather than changing the effect from one of benefit to one of harm, then it may be possible to adjust the result to reflect the impact in your patients. For example, if a treatment has been shown to be effective on a relatively fit study population, we might expect a greater effect to be observed on a very sick patient seen in practice. Similarly if a diagnostic test was assessed using a hospital population would it still be applicable in general practice?

Questions for assessing applicability

The assessment of both quality and applicability can be used to determine whether a study is worth reading in full. If a fundamental flaw is identified in the study design which means the results of the study cannot be trusted, there is little point in reading the full article. Similarly, if it is clear from the details presented in the study that the results cannot be applied to your patient population and/or the clinical setting, then there is no need to read further.

The assessment of applicability is not an exact science and requires some degree of subjectivity. Specific questions can help to ascertain the applicability of a study's results (CASP 2010). Unlike the quality assessment, the same questions can be used whatever type of question or study design is being appraised. Questions to consider when assessing applicability include the following:

- **What are the characteristics of the participants in the study?** Do they differ from the patients you see in practice? If so, do they differ on factors that could potentially affect the outcome of interest (consider age, co-morbidity, severity of condition, gender, etc.). Are the differences likely to affect the direction of the effect seen in the study or just the size of the effect?

- **Where has the study been conducted?** Is the study setting so different from yours that the results achieved in the study are unlikely to be achieved in your clinical setting? Again, are the differences likely to affect the direction of the effect seen in the study or just the magnitude of the effect?

- **Is it feasible to introduce the intervention or test described in the study?** Suppose the results of a research study into the care of patients with stroke suggest that patient outcomes are better when they are looked after in a specialist unit (i.e. one that requires certain types of equipment and staff with specialist training) rather than in a general ward. Such a change may not be possible on your unit. This does not mean that you should give up altogether (the issue should perhaps be referred to your unit manager); however, it does mean that you will need to look at other aspects of stroke management that are within the capacity of your team to deliver.

- **Have all the important outcomes been considered?** Have the researchers considered all the outcomes that are truly important to the patient and all those involved in their care and treatment planning? If not, how does this affect the interpretation of the results presented? Researchers often focus on outcome measures that are relatively quick and easy to measure, rather than those that are of practical importance. For example, surrogate outcomes, such as blood pressure, are often used to reflect the more clinically important outcomes, such as risk of heart attack. Surrogate outcomes are often used when the observation of a clinical outcome would require a long follow-up. However, when interpreting the findings from surrogate outcomes we have to be certain of the link between the surrogate and clinical outcome and whether its utility is well established.

- **Do any reported benefits outweigh the costs?** When thinking of the costs and benefits of the intervention or test, think beyond purely financial terms. In most situations doing something new or in a different way will involve stopping doing something else. The costs of 'stopping' need to be weighed up against the benefits of the proposed change. Where the costs are perceived by the patient and/or staff as being too high, the proposed change is unlikely to be accepted.

- **What are your patient's preferences?** Incorporating research evidence into practice should not mean ignoring patient preference. All patients are different and what one patient considers a reasonable intervention, treatment plan or outcome may be unacceptable to another. Forcing a patient to use the intervention indicated by evidence would be unethical and may be counterproductive.

Exercise

We encourage you to consolidate your learning by undertaking the worked exercises on the website.

Summary

In this chapter we have established why critical appraisal is necessary and important for evidence-based practice. The key principles of research design underpinning the assessment of a study have been outlined. Critical appraisal for evidence-based practice is a three-part process comprising assessment of the quality of the study, interpretation of the results, and assessment of the applicability of the findings to your patients in your setting. We have seen that it would be unrealistic to expect to find perfect research studies that match exactly a certain clinical context; the idea is to identify studies that can be applied to a specific context where the design is *good enough* for the results to be trusted. This chapter has provided examples of how this can be done for three different types of clinical question that require the use of different research designs. It is important to recognise that all three aspects of the critical appraisal process are interlinked. The quality and applicability aspects are probably the most important parts of critical appraisal to learn. Only you know the setting in which you wish to apply the results, and published studies very rarely assess their own quality, but it is becoming more common to publish study results in clinically useful forms. Chapter 8 describes how to use research evidence to inform clinical decisions for individual patients.

The tools in this chapter contain the basic questions necessary for assessing the quality of research studies in the practice environment. More sophisticated critical appraisal tools and techniques are available for people who are becoming more experienced or are doing critical appraisal on questions not covered in this chapter such as economic evaluations (Dumville & Soares 2009, Greenhalgh 2010). Presenting the results of critical appraisal to colleagues in a systematic way, making explicit the process used to come to these conclusions, is an important part of preparing for change (Melnyk 2005). The critical appraisal tools mentioned above provide a method for generating a summary of a study. Another way of doing this is to use critically appraised topics (CATs), which are one-page summaries of research papers. These were developed by the Centre for Evidence-Based Medicine in Oxford and examples of CATs can be accessed via their website (www.cebm.net). They also produce CATmaker software, which is a computer program that can be used to make CATs. Raw data from the study can be entered into the program to calculate some useful numbers for summarising the results in terms of effects on individual patients, e.g. the NNT.

It is important to recognise that critical appraisal is only one part of the evidence-based process and on its own will not result in improvements in the quality of care that you might want to achieve. It is therefore important that you take equal care to learn and practise the other stages in the process described in the other chapters of this manual. If the study is good enough to use and can be applied in the clinical setting of interest, the next step is to work out what to do about it. If a change in practice is required, how should that change be brought about? Simply telling colleagues that the evidence says they should be doing B rather than A has been demonstrated to be a rather ineffective change method (Mulhall 1999). Methods for increasing the chance of successfully changing practice are discussed in Chapters 9–10.

Acknowledgements

We give special thanks to Mark Newman, Tony Roberts, Faith Gibson and Anne-Marie Glenny whose contributions to previous editions have provided the foundation for this chapter.

References

Altman, D.G., 1998. Confidence intervals for the number needed to treat. Br. Med. J. 317, 1309–1312.

Arroll, B., Goodyear-Smith, F., Kerse, N., Fishman, T., Gunn, J., 2005. Effect of the addition of a "help" question to two screening questions on specificity for diagnosis of depression in general practice: diagnostic validity study. Br. Med. J. 331, 884–889.

Blaikie, N., 2000. Designing social research. Polity Press, Cambridge.

Bowling, A., 1997. Research methods in health: investigating health and health services. Open University Press, Buckingham.

Burns, N., Grove, S.K., 2001. The practice of nursing research: conduct, critique and utilization, fourth ed. W B Saunders, Philadelphia.

CASP Critical Appraisal Skills Programme. 2004. 12 questions to help you make sense of a cohort study. Public Health Resource Unit, England. Available online at: http://www.sph.nhs.uk/sph-files/cohort%2012%20questions.pdf.

CASP Critical Appraisal Skills Programme, 2006a. 10 questions to help you make sense of randomised controlled trials. Public Health Resource Unit, England. Available online at: http://www.sph.nhs.uk/sph-files/rct%20appraisal%20tool.pdf.

CASP Critical Appraisal Skills Programme, 2006b. 12 questions to help you make sense of a diagnostic test study. Public Health Resource Unit, England. Available online at: http://www.sph.nhs.uk/sph-files/Diagnostic%20Tests%2012%20Questions.pdf.

CASP Critical Appraisal Skills Programme. 2006c. 11 questions to help you make sense of a case control study. Public Health Resource Unit, England. Available online at: http://www.sph.nhs.uk/sph-files/Case%20Control%2011%20Questions.pdf.

CASP Critical Appraisal Skills Programme, 2010. Available online at: http://www.sph.nhs.uk/what-we-do/public-health-workforce/resources/critical-appraisals-skills-programme (accessed November 2010).

Chalmers, I., Altman, D.G., 1995. Systematic reviews. BMJ Publishing, London.

Cullinan, P., 2005. Evidence-based health-care: systematic reviews. In: Bowling, A., Ebrahim, S. (Eds.), Handbook of health research methods: investigation, measurement and analysis. Open University Press, Buckingham, pp. 47–61.

Dumville, J., Soares, M., 2009. The economics of clinical decision making. In: Thompson, C., Dowding, D. (Eds.), Essential decision making and clinical judgement for nurses. Churchill Livingstone, London, pp. 197–216.

Evans, D., Pearson, A., 2001. Systematic reviews: gatekeepers of nursing knowledge. J. Clin. Nurs. 10, 593–599.

French, P., 2002. What is the evidence on evidence-based nursing? An epistemological concern. J. Adv. Nurs. 37 (3), 250–257.

Gardner, M., Altman, D.G., 1986. Confidence intervals rather than P values: estimation rather than hypothesis testing. Br. Med. J. 292, 746–750.

Gray, J.A.M., 1997. Evidence-based health-care: how to make health policy and management decisions. Churchill Livingstone, Edinburgh.

Greenhalgh, T., 1997. How to read a paper: assessing the methodological quality of published papers. Br. Med. J. 315, 305–308.

Greenhalgh, T., 2010. How to read a paper, the basics of evidence-based medicine, fourth ed. John Wiley and Sons Ltd, Chichester, pp. 149–162.

Guyatt, G., Rennie, D., Meade, M.O., Cook, D.J., 2008. Users' guides to the medical literature: a manual for evidence-based clinical practice, second ed. McGraw-Hill, New York.

Johnston, L., 2005. Critically appraising quantitative evidence. In: Melnyk, B.M., Fineout-Overholt, E. (Eds.), Evidence-based practice in nursing and health-care: a guide to best practice. Lippincott Williams and Wilkins, Philadelphia, pp. 79–125.

Kirkwood, B., 1988. Essentials of medical statistics. Blackwell Science, Oxford.

Last, J.M., 1988. A dictionary of epidemiology. Oxford University Press, Oxford.

Laupacis, A., Sackett, D.L., Roberts, R.S., 1988. An assessment of clinically useful measures of the consequences of treatment. N. Engl. J. Med. 318 (26), 1728–1733.

Laupacis, A., Wells, G., Richardson, S., Tugwell, P., 1994. Users' guides to the medical literature. V. How to use an article about prognosis. J. Am. Med. Assoc. 272, 234–237.

Lijmer, J.G., Mol, B.W., Heisterkamp, S., Bonsel, G.J., Prins, M.H., van der Meulen, J.H., et al., 1999. Empirical evidence of design-related bias in studies of diagnostic tests. J. Am. Med. Assoc. 282, 1061–1066.

Mant, J., 1999a. Studies assessing diagnostic tests. In: Dawes, M., Davies, P., Gray, A., Mant, J., Seers, J., Snowball, R. (Eds.), Evidence-based practice: a primer for health-care professionals. Churchill Livingstone, London, pp. 59–69.

Mant, J., 1999b. Case control studies. In: Dawes, M., Davies, P., Gray, A., Mant, J., Seers, J., Snowball, R. (Eds.), Evidence-based practice: a primer for health-care professionals. Churchill Livingstone, London, pp. 73–85.

Mant, J., 1999c. Is this test effective? In: Dawes, M., Davies, P., Gray, A., Mant, J., Seers, J., Snowball, R. (Eds.), Evidence-based practice: a primer for health care professionals. Churchill Livingstone, London, pp. 133–157.

Martin, R.M., 2005. Epidemiological study designs for health-care research and evaluation. In: Bowling, A., Ebrahim, S. (Eds.), Handbook of health research methods: investigation, measurement and analysis. Open University Press, Buckingham, pp. 98–163.

Matthews, J.N.S., 2000. An introduction to randomized controlled clinical trials. Arnold, London.

Melnyk, B.M., 2005. Creating a vision: motivating a change to evidence-based practice in individuals and organizations. In: Melnyk, B.M., Fineout-Over-holt, E. (Eds.), Evidence-based practice in nursing and healthcare: a guide to best practice. Lippincott Williams and Wilkins, Philadelphia, pp. 443–455.

Moher, D., Jadad, E.R., Nichol, G., Penman, M., Tugwell, P., Walsh, S., 1995. Assessing the quality of randomised controlled trials: an annotated bibliography of scales and checklists. Control. Clin. Trials 16, 62–73.

Moore, A., McQuay, H., 2000. Bias. Bandolier 7 (10), 1–5.

Mulhall, A., 1999. Creating change in practice. In: Mulhall, A., Le May, A. Nursing research: dissemination and implementation. Churchill Livingstone, Edinburgh, pp. 151–175.

O'Rourke, A., 2005. Critical appraisal. In: Bowling, A., Ebrahim, S. (Eds.) Handbook of health research methods: investigation, measurement and analysis. Open University Press, Buckingham, pp. 62–84.

Oxman, A.D., Sackett, D.L., Guyatt, G.H., the Evidence-Based Medicine Working Group, 1993. How to get started. Based on the Users' Guides to Evidence-Based Medicine and reproduced with permission from Journal of the American Medical Association 270 (17), 2093–2095.

Sackett, D.L., Rosenberg, W.M.C., Muir Gray, J.A., Haynes, R.B., Richardson, W.S., 1996. Evidence based medicine: what it is and what it isn't. Br. Med. J. 312, 71–72.

Sackett, D., Strauss, S., Scott Richardson, W., Rosenberg, W., Haynes, R., 2000. Evidence-based medicine: how to practise and teach evidence-based medicine, second ed. Churchill Livingstone, Edinburgh.

Scurr, J.H., Machin, S.J., Bailey-King, S., Mackie, I.J., McDonald, S., Coleridge Smith, P.D., 2001. Frequency and prevention of symptomless deep-vein thrombosis in long-haul flights: a randomized trial. Lancet 357, 1485–1489.

Sim, J., Wright, C., 2000. Basic elements of research design. In: Sim, J., Wright, C. (Eds.), Research in health-care: concepts, designs and methods. Nelson Thornes, Cheltenham.

Stevens, K.R., 2005. Critically appraising knowledge for clinical decision making. In: Melnyk, B.M., Fineout-Overholt, E. (Eds.), Evidence-based practice in nursing and health-care: a guide to best practice. Lippincott Williams and Wilkins, Philadelphia, pp. 73–78.

Summerskill, W.S.M., 2000. Hierarchy of evidence. In: McGovern, D.B.P., Valori, R.M., Summerskill, W.S.M., Levi, M. (Eds.), Evidence-based medicine. BIOS Scientific Publishers, Oxford, pp. 14–16.

von Ungern-Sternberg, B.S., Boda, K., Chambers, N.A., Rebmann, C., Johnson, C., Sly, P.D., et al., 2010. Risk assessment for respiratory complications in paediatric anaesthesia: a prospective cohort study. Lancet 376, 773–783.

Further reading

Internet resources

There are numerous websites that contain materials for critical appraisal. However, these sites often change their website address and new sites are opening up all the time. The Centre for Evidence Based Medicine at Oxford has a number of useful resources found at www.cebm.net as does www.jamaevidence.com but the latter requires a subscription.

Books

Crombie, I.K., 1996. The pocket guide to critical appraisal. BMJ Publishing, London.

Greenhalgh, T., 2010. How to read a paper, fourth ed. BMJ Books, John Wiley and Sons Ltd, Chichester.

Melnyk, B.M., Fineout-Overholt, E., 2005. Evidence-based practice in nursing and health-care: a guide to best practice. Lippincott Williams and Wilkins, Philadelphia.

Ogier, M.E., 2002. Reading research, how to make research more approachable, third ed. Baillière Tindall, London.

Sackett, D., Strauss, S., Scott Richardson, W., Rosenberg, W., Haynes, R., 2000. Evidence-based medicine: how to practise and teach evidence-based medicine, second ed. Churchill Livingstone, Edinburgh.

CHAPTER

Using evidence from systematic reviews

Rosalind L Smyth and Leanne V Jones

KEY POINTS

- Systematic reviews use rigorous methods to reduce bias and can provide reliable summaries of relevant research evidence.

- Because systematic reviews include a comprehensive search strategy, appraisal and synthesis of research evidence, they can be used as shortcuts in the evidence-based process.

- The Cochrane Library, which is updated monthly, electronically includes a database of up-to-date systematic reviews from across the whole of health care.

- Critical appraisal of systematic reviews is necessary to ensure that they have been conducted to rigorous standards.

- Meta-analysis is a statistical technique used in systematic reviews. It can answer the questions 'does this intervention have a beneficial effect?' and if so, 'what is the size of that effect?

What are systematic reviews?

Reviews of healthcare literature take many shapes and forms depending on the type and expertise of the audience to which they are addressed. They may include chapters in textbooks, reports to expert committees and 'state of the art' reviews for clinical journals. The main purpose of these reviews is to bring their audience rapidly up to speed with the current information in specific clinical areas.

It is partly because of the explosion in information technology that we have come to rely increasingly on reviews. Healthcare professionals at every stage of their career development often feel overwhelmed by the magnitude of literature available to them. Evidence-based health care offers some solutions to this problem (McKibbon et al 2005). It is because health professionals are inundated by so many publications that they have come to rely on summaries of the evidence in the form of reviews. Many of these review articles are well researched, beautifully illustrated and highly entertaining and informative. However, as 'bottom line' summaries of which treatments, diagnostic tests, etc., are effective, they may be misleading. One reason for this is that reviews are often written by acknowledged experts, who are likely to have already formed an opinion about what works, and who may not review the evidence in an unbiased manner. Another reason is that writing reviews is not always regarded as the most important academic activity and less time is devoted to it than, for example, writing up original research. So those writing the reviews may cut corners and rehash something they have written previously, rather than undertaking an exhaustive search and critical appraisal of all the evidence.

Let us take the example quoted by Professor Paul Knipschild in the book *Systematic Reviews* (Knipschild 1995). He describes how the distinguished biochemist Linus Pauling, writing in his book *How to Live Long and Feel Better* (Pauling 1986), quoted more than 30 trials that supported his contention that vitamin C could prevent the common cold. Knipschild and colleagues then went on to do their own 'systematic review' which showed that even large doses of vitamin C cannot prevent a cold, although they may slightly decrease its duration and severity. A critical review of what Pauling had written showed that he had omitted a number of important studies which did not support the contention that he so enthusiastically proposed. There are now many examples that have shown that unsystematic or narrative reviews do not routinely incorporate all relevant up-to-date scientific evidence.

This shortcoming has led to the notion that reviews need to be performed systematically. This means that the same rigour that we expect of people undertaking primary research should be demanded of reviewers undertaking this very important task of 'research synthesis' or 'secondary research'. You will have seen from Chapter 5 that in studies such as randomised controlled trials (RCTs) and diagnostic tests, the study can be designed so that bias is reduced or eliminated. Strategies such as blinding (or masking) investigators and participants in clinical trials to whether they are in the experimental or the control group may be introduced to prevent the human element of bias.

In the same way, strategies can be introduced to the reviewing process to eliminate the human element of bias caused, for example, by the reviewer having a strong opinion about whether the treatment under review works. The methodology of a systematic review is outlined in Box 6.1. The research needs to start with a protocol which first of all states clearly the hypothesis or question that the investigator is addressing. In Chapter 2 we have already discussed the importance of formulating an appropriate question. A systematic reviewer needs to define their question very precisely as everything else in the methodology will flow from this. Systematic reviews can address a range of questions relating to the effectiveness of an intervention, the prognosis of a particular condition, the accuracy of a diagnostic test or the qualitative experience of a group of patients.

The search itself should be comprehensive, including not only electronic databases (e.g. MEDLINE) but also, where possible, sources of unpublished studies. This may seem odd, but there

---

BOX 6.1 How to conduct a systematic review

1. State objectives and hypotheses.
2. Outline eligibility criteria, stating types of study, types of participants, types of interventions and outcomes to be examined.
3. Perform a comprehensive search of all relevant sources for potentially eligible studies.
4. Examine the studies to decide eligibility (if possible with two independent reviewers).
5. Construct a table describing the characteristics of the included studies.
6. Assess methodological quality of included studies (if possible with two independent reviewers).
7. Extract data (with a second investigator if possible) with involvement of investigators if necessary.
8. Analyse results of included studies, using statistical synthesis of data (meta-analysis), if appropriate.
9. Prepare a report of review, stating aims, materials and methods and describing results and conclusions.

---

is a phenomenon known as 'publication bias': for any intervention, there may be studies that do not show a clear benefit of the intervention compared with the control group and these studies are less likely to be published (Decullier et al 2005, Decullier & Chapius 2007, Easterbrook et al 1991). Excluding unpublished studies from systematic reviews may bias the results of the review towards studies in which a benefit of the intervention was observed. Unpublished studies can be retrieved in a number of ways, none of which is perfect. One way of doing this is to search for abstracts of studies presented at conferences, available in the abstract books of relevant international conferences. Another common feature of systematic reviews, which may impair their quality, is that they may exclude study reports that are not published in English thus ignoring potentially important information. An example is the field of complementary medicine; many studies of acupuncture are published in non-English language journals, particularly those from China (McCarney et al 2003).

The next step in the review is to decide what studies should be included. This should be done according to rigorous inclusion and exclusion criteria so that systematic bias can be avoided. These criteria should be stated in the review methods in the form of: the types of study design, the types of participants, the types of interventions and the types of outcomes. For example, Poustie et al (1999) have published a review on the Cochrane Library entitled 'Oral protein calorie supplementation for children with chronic disease'. The types of participants were stated as children aged 1–16 years with any defined chronic disease. Trials undertaken in children suffering from malnutrition who did not have an associated disease were not included.

These clearly stated eligibility criteria can then be applied to all the studies retrieved from the search. Again, to reduce bias it is best if more than one reviewer can do this, working independently of each other. The reviewers can then compare which studies they have independently included. They should have previously worked out a mechanism for deciding what to do if there are differences between their lists of included studies. This may mean involving a third reviewer. In the review of oral protein calorie supplementation, the search identified a very large number of studies conducted in children suffering from the effects of famine. The question of whether this intervention is effective in children with severe undernutrition in this setting is a very important one, but was not the question addressed in Poustie and colleagues' review and thus these studies were excluded.

Having decided which studies are eligible for inclusion, the reviewers need to tabulate their characteristics. This description should include the study methods, details of the participants, the precise nature of the interventions and the outcomes measured. You will notice that, in tabulating the study characteristics, the reviewers are describing the studies under the headings by which they have determined whether or not the study is eligible for inclusion in the review. For this reason, it may be helpful if steps 4 and 5 (Box 6.1) are done together. When reviewers are trying to determine whether a study is eligible for inclusion in a review, in many cases it is very obvious whether this is the case or not.

However, by tabulating the characteristics of all studies where one or more reviewers think the study may be included, it will soon become apparent whether the inclusion criteria have been fulfilled. The final table of included studies, which all reviewers have agreed, will appear in the review and the readers can judge if the reviewers got it right. For each study excluded, the reviewers need to state, in the review, the reason for this exclusion, and again the reader can judge whether this is valid.

For example, Table 6.1 provides details of a study by Kalnins et al (2005) which was included in the review of oral protein calorie supplementation. This study included children and adults with cystic fibrosis over the age of 10, but the review addressed children only. However, the reviewers were able to obtain summary data on the children included in the trial by contacting the investigators in the original study. All the outcomes evaluated in the trial are listed and those which are evaluated in the review are asterisked. When reading a review, examination of the 'Characteristics of included studies' can help the reader to decide whether the review is applicable to their question. The reader may have in mind a particular age of patient or a specific type of intervention. If none of the studies has included this age of patient or type of intervention, then it is less likely that the review will be relevant.

The protocol should describe how the quality (risk of bias) of the included studies will be assessed and how the data will be extracted and analysed. Again, it is best if these steps are performed by more than one person. The quality (risk of bias) of the studies should be assessed using an appropriate checklist or tool. The use of tools which encompass a numerical summary score are not recommended (Higgins et al 2011). There are many checklists now available for the assessment of RCTs and other study designs. In Cochrane systematic reviews, studies are graded according to their risk of bias (Higgins et al 2011). Each individual study is assessed in order to judge whether it has a low, high or unclear risk of bias. It may be possible to separately analyse only the studies with a low risk of bias. In a systematic review examining the effects of omega 3 fatty acids in the prevention and treatment of cardiovascular disease (Hooper et al 2004),

TABLE 6.1 CHARACTERISTICS OF INCLUDED STUDY (© COCHRANE LIBRARY, REPRODUCED WITH PERMISSION)

Study	Methods	Participants	Interventions	Outcomes
Kalnins et al 2005	Quasi-randomised, parallel design	Cystic fibrosis patients aged > 10 years, <90% ideal weight for height, or greater than 5% reduction in ideal weight for height over previous 3 months	High-calorie drinks to increase energy intake by 20% of predicted energy needs. Control group received nutritional counselling to increase energy intake by 20% of predicted energy needs by normal diet. Study period: 3 months	Z scores for weight and height;* percentage ideal weight for height;* anthropometric measures;* pulmonary function;* energy and nutrient intake;* faecal balance studies

* Protocol-defined outcome measures.

Data from Kalnins et al (2005).

a pooled analysis of all the studies indicated no reduction in the risk of cardiovascular disease. A separate analysis, retaining only studies at low risk of bias, again suggested no significant effect of omega 3 fats. Since the results of this analysis are the same as those obtained when all studies were analysed, we can be reassured that the results were not affected by including the higher risk of bias studies. This is known as a 'sensitivity analysis'. Methodological assessment of quality of included studies is very important in a review, but it needs to be judged in an unbiased way.

The next steps in the review process are to extract the data and analyse them. When the reviewers stated their outcomes, they would have provided some indication of what measures they expected to find. The measures used in individual studies will be further described in the table of study characteristics. For example, in Table 6.1 it will be seen that in the trial by Kalnins et al (2005), there were various measures of nutritional status, pulmonary function and energy intake. In extracting the data, the reviewers need to examine exactly what these measures are, for each trial, for the outcomes in which they are interested. They should draw up their own data extraction form, listing the measures made in each trial. In some situations statistical analysis of the results may not be possible. For example, slightly different measurements of outcomes may have been made in each of the included trials and because of this they cannot be combined as one summary outcome measure. This is referred to as heterogeneity (explained more fully later in the chapter). In this situation, reviewers should summarise the results of the individual studies, in narrative or tabular form, in the review. If a meta-analysis (statistical synthesis of the results of the individual studies) has not been possible, the results of the review (which should be the best possible summary of the evidence) are still robust.

Meta-analysis will be explained in detail later in this chapter. Essentially, in the analysis, sensible comparisons should be made and the results should be expressed in a way that is easy to understand. A common mistake is to confuse 'no evidence of effect' with 'evidence of no effect' (Schünemann et al 2011). A review may conclude that there is no evidence to show that a treatment works, but this does not mean that the treatment does not work. Results from analysis of specific groups of patients (known as 'subgroups') should be interpreted with caution. The conclusions should be supported by the results and extravagant claims avoided.

By writing a protocol before they start the review, the reviewers are ensuring that their methods will not be influenced by prior knowledge of the studies that they are going to encounter. The methodology is made clear and if there are any potential sources of bias, it is available for people to examine externally. It is this methodology that largely distinguishes a systematic review from a narrative or literature review.

Cochrane Systematic Reviews

In most descriptions of evidence-based practice, a four-step approach is proposed (Box 6.2). It will be apparent from the previous discussion that if you are able to directly access a systematic review which addresses the question posed, the systematic review would have already performed steps 2 and 3. Systematic reviews are, therefore, a 'shortcut', which the evidence-based practitioner can use to answer specific questions relating to clinical management. The laborious tasks of searching and critical appraisal will already have been done by the reviewer. However, to be confident of this process, one would need to be reassured that the systematic reviews being accessed were of high quality. In the end, rather than accessing databases of primary research studies such as CINAHL or MEDLINE, would it not be much more convenient to access the database of systematic reviews? This is, in effect, what the Cochrane Database of Systematic Reviews, which is contained in

---

BOX 6.2 Four steps in an evidence-based approach

1. Ask a clinically relevant question.
2. Search for the best available external evidence.
3. Critically appraise that evidence for its validity and relevance.
4. Apply the evidence in clinical practice.

the Cochrane Library, provides. The Cochrane Library has been referred to previously but here we shall discuss its merits as a source of systematic reviews.

There are two main problems with systematic reviews published in paper journals. The first is that in reviewing the evidence, one wishes to be assured that the systematic review is up to date. In a paper journal, a systematic review can only be current up to the date of publication. This means that studies published subsequently will not have been included and these may change the results and conclusions of the systematic review. Secondly, systematic reviews require a lot of work, particularly in the meticulous searching for appropriate studies and their critical appraisal. It would be very disheartening indeed to discover just before you were due to submit a manuscript of a systematic review for publication that you had been 'pipped to the post' by somebody doing the same systematic review.

Both of these problems have been addressed by the Cochrane Collaboration. This is an international body of researchers who have responded to the challenge of the British epidemiologist Archie Cochrane. It was he who observed that 'it is surely a great criticism of our profession that we have not organised a critical summary by specialty or subspecialty adapted periodically of all relevant randomised controlled trials' (Cochrane 1979). Systematic reviews published on the Cochrane Library are regularly updated as new evidence becomes available. Duplication of effort is avoided as individual review groups within the Collaboration publish the titles of all systematic reviews as soon as the review process has started. The other important advantage of Cochrane Systematic Reviews is that they are of high quality. For example, Jadad et al (2000) have published an evaluation of reviews and meta-analyses of treatments used in asthma. Of the 50 reviews they included, 40 were found to have serious or extensive methodological flaws. They found that Cochrane Reviews had higher overall quality scores than those published in peer review journals.

The methodology for Cochrane Reviews has been developed by the Cochrane Collaboration and follows the same steps outlined in Box 6.1. The protocol of the review is published first of all on the Cochrane Library so that readers of the Library can examine the proposed methodology, before the results of the review are available. The coverage of the Cochrane Library does not extend to the whole of health care as yet. However, Issue 6, 2010 of the Cochrane Database of Systematic Reviews contained 4281 completed systematic reviews. We searched the Cochrane Library using the free text term nurs* combined with the MeSH descriptor 'nursing' and achieved hits on 178 of these 4281 reviews, so many of them are relevant to nursing practice. Clearly, if one is able to identify a systematic review on the Cochrane Library that addresses the question of interest, this is a much quicker process than starting with other electronic databases. One can also be confident that all the relevant clinical studies will have been included.

Critical appraisal of systematic reviews

Box 6.3 shows a checklist adapted from the Critical Appraisal Skills Programme (CASP) 2010 for assessment of review articles. This checklist should clearly enable the reader to distinguish

---

BOX 6.3 Checklist for appraising systematic reviews

1. Did the review ask a clearly focused question?
2. Did the review include the right type of study?
3. Did the review try to identify all relevant studies?
4. Did the review assess the quality of the included studies?
5. If the results of the studies have been combined, was it reasonable to do so?
6. How have the results been presented and what is the main result?
7. How precise are these results?
8. Can the results be applied to the local population?
9. Were all important outcomes considered?
10. Should policy or practice change as a result of the evidence contained in this review?

(CASP checklist "10 questions to help you make sense of reviews" reproduced with permission from Solutions for Public Health, © *Public Health Resource Unit, England* (2006). All rights reserved.)

between narrative and systematic reviews, but should also enable the reader to assess the quality of systematic reviews and the rigour of the methodology. The latter point is particularly important as there is now evidence of considerable variation in quality of systematic reviews. The term 'systematic review' may have been applied to something inferior, in order to give it legitimacy.

When you have completed reading this chapter, we recommend that you undertake the critical appraisal exercise.

Understanding meta-analysis

Like all quantitative studies, systematic reviews often include a statistical analysis. This involves combining the data from the included studies in a process referred to as 'meta-analysis'. This analysis may be very powerful. The individual studies that make up a review are, on their own, often small and unableto detect whether or not a treatment is effective but when the data from a number of similar small studies are combined, valid conclusions may be drawn. Often the terms 'meta-analysis' and 'systematic review' are used interchangeably. This is inappropriate because, as can be seen from Box 6.1, meta-analysis is simply one of the final steps in what must be a rigorous process. Statistical aggregation of the data in a meta-analysis does not mean that the individual studies included in the meta-analysiswere reviewed systematically or appropriately. The most important part of the process is the one that we have already described, which refers to all the elements in the review process set up to prevent bias.

The Cochrane logo (Fig. 6.1) is a stylised diagram of a meta-analysis from a systematic review. This systematic review included data from seven RCTs, which investigated the effect of corticosteroids administered to pregnant women who were about to deliver prematurely. The outcome examined was the survival of their infant. The vertical line is where these results would be expected to cluster if this treatment had a similar effect to the control group (placebo or no treatment) and each horizontal line represents the results of one trial. The shorter the line, the more certain the result, because the 95% confidence intervals are narrow. If the horizontal line lies entirely to the left

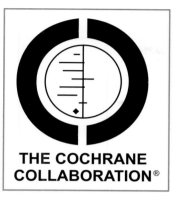

Figure 6.1 The Cochrane Collaboration logo, indicating a meta-analysis of seven randomised controlled trials comparing corticosteroids versus no corticosteroids in pregnant women about to deliver prematurely. (© The Cochrane Collaboration. HYPERLINK "http://www .cochrane.org" www.cochrane.org. Reproduced with permission.)

of the vertical line, the treatment has shown significant benefit. If it touches or crosses the vertical line then clear benefit was not demonstrated in that trial. If the horizontal line were to lie entirely to the right of the vertical line, then more babies would have died in the treatment group than in the control group, i.e. the treatment would have been harmful. The trial at the top of the diagram was performed in 1972 and did show benefit, but the four subsequent trials did not. The sixth trial did show benefit and the seventh did not. On a simple 'vote count' (five of the trials showed no benefit) one might be persuaded not to use this intervention. However, when a systematic review was performed with meta-analysis and first reported in 1989 (Crowley 1996), this showed that corticosteroids administered to pregnant women reduced the odds of their babies dying by between 30% and 50%. This meta-analysis is indicated by the solid diamond at the bottom of the diagram.

Meta-analysis can answer two main questions about a treatment: 'Does this intervention have a beneficial (or harmful) effect?' and if so 'What is the size of that effect?' We will consider this with reference to specific examples. First, there are some terms used in expressing results that need to be explained. The first is known as the 'relative risk' (or risk ratio). The risk (or proportion, probability or rate) is the ratio

TABLE 6.2 TABLE SHOWING HOW RESULTS OF A PROSPECTIVE STUDY ARE REPRESENTED

		Group 1	Group 2	Total
Outcome present	Yes	a	b	a + b
	No	c	d	c + d
	Total	a + c	b + d	n

of people with an event in a group compared with the total in that group. In Table 6.2, the risk of the outcome being present in group 1 is:

$$\frac{a}{a+c}$$

In 2007, a clinical trial published by Nelson et al (2007) compared two types of bandaging for the treatment of venous ulcers. One was multi-component high-compression bandaging, which is widely used in the UK, and the other was single component low-compression bandaging, used in standard practice in mainland Europe and Australia. The outcome that we will consider is complete healing of the ulcer within the trial period. There were 117 patients in the high-compression bandaging group and 128 in the low-compression group. Table 6.3 shows the numbers in each group which had complete healing. So the risk of complete ulcer healing in the high-compression group is 78/117 and the risk of complete healing in the low-pressure group is 63/128.

In a clinical trial, the relative risk is the ratio of the risk in the intervention group to the risk in the control group. For this trial, the relative risk is:

$$\frac{78/117}{63/128} = \frac{0.67}{0.49} = 1.36$$

If the risk in the treatment group is the same as that in the comparison group, the ratio will be 1. This means that there is no difference between the treatment and the comparison group.

The 'odds ratio' is the ratio of the odds of an event in the treatment group compared to the odds of an event in the comparison

TABLE 6.3 RELATION BETWEEN COMPLETE ULCER HEALING AND HIGH-COMPRESSION OR LOW-COMPRESSION BANDAGING

		High compression		Low compression		Total
Complete healing	Yes	78	a	b	63	141
	No	39	c	d	65	104
	Total	117			128	245

Data from Nelson et al 2007.

group. The odds are the ratio of the number of people in a group with an event compared to the number without an event. So, looking again at Table 6.2, the odds of a patient in group 1 having the outcome present are:

a/c

In the Nelson trial, the odds of complete ulcer healing in the high-compression group are:

78/39 = 2.0

In the low-compression group, the odds of complete ulcer healing are:

63/65 = 0.97

The odds ratio of complete ulcer healing in the two groups is:

2.0/0.97 = 2.1

If the odds of the event in the treatment group are the same as those in the comparison group then the odds ratio is again 1. That is, there is no difference between the treatment and comparison groups.

Where the outcome of interest is rare, in Table 6.2, a will be very small and a/(a + c) will be approximately equal to a/c. Similarly b/(b + d) will approximately equal b/d. Thus, when the outcome is rare, the risks of the outcomes in the two groups will be very similar to the odds of the outcomes in the two groups and the relative risks will be very similar to the odds ratios.

Ninety-five percent confidence intervals are an expression of how precise the estimate of the odds ratio or relative risk is. This gives an estimate of the range to 95% certainty that the true result for odds ratio or relative risk lies within the range stated.

Let us consider now a systematic review by O'Meara et al (2009), which assessed the effectiveness of compression bandaging or stockings in treatment of venous leg ulceration. Included in this review was the comparison between high-compression (four-component bandage) and low-compression bandaging (single component), which we have referred to previously. Another comparison included within this review was a comparison between elastic multi-component bandages and inelastic multi-component bandages (three components). Two trials that made this comparison were found. This meta-analysis is illustrated in Table 6.4. The ratios shown in the column labelled '3 component (elastic)' indicate the number of patients in the experimental group with complete healing compared with the total number of patients in that group. These risks are shown both for each individual study and, at the bottom, for the two studies combined. The term 'risk', as used here, is misleading, because the effect of ulcer healing is beneficial, but I have retained it for consistency. The combined result gives a relative risk (or risk ratio) of 1.83. This represents the relative benefit increase for healing for the elastic multi-component bandaging. You will recall that if the two treatments were equally effective, this ratio should be 1. Instead, it is 1.83. This means there is an 83% relative benefit increase for healing in the elastic multi-component bandaging group. O'Meara et al (2009) calculated the 95% confidence intervals for the relative risks. For this relative benefit increase of 83%, the 95% confidence intervals were 1.26 to 2.67. This is a very wide range, within which the true benefit increase is estimated to lie 95% of the time. However, even the lowest estimate of 26% indicates clear benefit of the elastic multi-component bandaging over the inelastic multi-component bandaging, and this is a statistically significant result.

TABLE 6.4 COMPRESSION FOR VENOUS LEG ULCERS. THE COMPARISON SHOWN IS FOR THREE COMPONENTS INCLUDING ELASTIC BANDAGE VERSUS THREE COMPONENTS INELASTIC BANDAGE (RR AND 95% CONFIDENCE INTERVAL). THE OUTCOME IS PATIENTS/LIMBS WITH COMPLETE HEALING DURING TRIAL (VARYING LENGTHS) (COPYRIGHT COCHRANE LIBRARY, WITH PERMISSION)

Review: Compression for venous leg ulcers

Comparison: 3 components including elastic bandage vs 3 components including inelastic bandage (RR and 95% Confidence Interval)

Outcome: Patients/limbs with complete healing during trial

Study or subgroup	3 components (elastic)		3 components (inelastic)		Weight	Risk Ratio M-H, Fixed, 95% CI	Risk Ratio M-H, Fixed, 95% CI
	Events	Total	Events	Total			
Callam 1992	35	65	19	67	73.3%	1.90 [1.22, 2.95]	
Gould 1998	11	19	7	20	26.7%	1.65 [0.81, 3.36]	
Total (95%CL)		84		87	100.0%	1.83 [1.26, 2.67]	
Total events	46		26				

Heterogeneity: Chi^2 = 0.10, df = 1 (P = 0.75); I^2 = 0%

Test for overall effect: Z = 3.16 (P = 0.002)

Data with permission from O'Meara et al (2009).

In the text of their review, O'Meara et al (2009) chose to express their results as relative risk, rather than odds ratios. However, in Table 6.5, the right-hand column demonstrates the odds ratio with 95% confidence interval:

2.85 [1.52, 5.35]

Now look at the final column. You will see a number of 'blobs' bisected by horizontal lines. Reading the figures along the bottom axis, the position of the blob represents the odds ratio for each individual trial.

The horizontal line represents the 95% confidence interval of the individual trial. In this situation if both the odds ratio and

TABLE 6.5 COMPRESSION FOR VENOUS LEG ULCERS. THE COMPARISON SHOWN IS FOR THREE COMPONENTS INCLUDING ELASTIC BANDAGE VERSUS THREE COMPONENTS INCLUDING INELASTIC BANDAGE (OR AND 95% CONFIDENCE INTERVAL). THE OUTCOME IS PATIENTS/LIMBS WITH COMPLETE HEALING DURING TRIAL (COPYRIGHT COCHRANE LIBRARY, WITH PERMISSION)

Study or subgroup	3 components (elastic)		3 components (inelastic)		Weight	Odds Ratio M-H, Fixed, 95% CI	Odds Ratio M-H, Fixed, 95% CI
	Events	Total	Events	Total			
Callam 1992	35	65	19	67	75%	2.95 [1.43, 6.06]	
Gould 1998	11	19	7	20	25%	2.55 [0.70, 9.31]	
Total (95%CL)		84		87	100.0%	2.85 [1.52, 5.35]	
Total events	46		26				

Heterogeneity: Chi^2 = 0.04, df = 1 (P = 0.85); I^2 = 0%
Test for overall effect: Z = 3.26 (P = 0.001)
Data with permission from O'Meara et al (2009).

the 95% confidence interval lie entirely to the right of the vertical line at 1, it means there is a statistically significant benefit, in this case of elastic multi-component bandages compared to inelastic multi-component bandages, for the outcome being examined (complete healing of the ulcer in the trial period). If one looks at the two individual trials, it will be seen that this applies to only one trial (Callam). In the other trial (Gould) the horizontal line crosses the vertical line of 1. This means that, although the odds ratio lies to the right of the line (Gould), the 95% confidence intervals include the line, so it is possible that the true result is 1 or even slightly less than 1, which means that there is no significant benefit. However, if the results from both trials are combined, the total result shown by the diamond at the bottom, where the 'blob' lies to the right of 1, indicates that the combined result is significant. The odds ratio of 2.85 suggests a large benefit of elastic multi-component bandaging over inelastic multi-component bandaging. O'Meara et al

(2009) chose to express their results as relative risks rather than odds ratios, because their outcome of interest (complete ulcer healing) was not rare in either group. You will recall from the previous discussion that relative risks and odds ratios are only similar if the outcome is rare. The authors felt that to quote odds ratios would give an inflated impression of the magnitude of the effect.

In a meta-analysis, each study does not make an equal contribution to the pooled estimate. Rather, studies are given a 'weight', specified as a percentage, to reflect the amount of information that they contain. The more informative the study, the more weight it is given and the greater its contribution to the pooled estimate. The contribution to the pooled estimate of each of the studies is shown in the column labelled Weight %.

It is important when interpreting a meta-analysis to look for evidence of heterogeneity. Any differences between the individual trials in terms of patients, interventions and outcomes (clinical heterogeneity) or in terms of the methods used in the individual trials (methodological heterogeneity) need to be considered. If you consider that the differences between trials are too great, then it may not be appropriate to pool the data in a meta-analysis. Heterogeneity can be assessed visually by examining the meta-analysis and also with the aid of statistical tests (Chi-squared; I-squared). The first step in assessing possible heterogeneity is to see if the results of the individual trials within the meta-analysis (forest plot) are generally overlapping and not scattered. The next step is to look at the value of Chi-squared (Chi^2). A non-significant result is indicated by a P value greater than 0.10 and indicates that heterogeneity is not present. However, this needs to be interpreted together with the I-squared test. This is because the Chi^2 test is not a robust test when the number of trials in an analysis is small and may give a non-significant result even when important heterogeneity is present. Finally, the I-squared statistic quantifies the amount of heterogeneity. If the I-squared exceeds 50%, then heterogeneity may be substantial.

How can systematic reviews inform practice?

Let us suppose that you are a practice nurse working in a busy inner-city practice. There are high rates of unemployment and social deprivation within your practice population. You are concerned to find that three men, all in their early 40s, have recently died from acute myocardial infarction. All three men were on your GP's list, but none had attended the surgery for the last 5 years. All were smokers.

These tragedies have prompted you to consider setting up a 'well man' clinic. The aim of the clinic would be to identify men with risk factors for cardiovascular disease, and try to implement lifestyle changes which may reduce these risks. You plan to review all men on the practice list aged 40–60 in the first instance. Because of the large number of people that this will involve, you will have a limited time for detailed discussions with each individual. You are in a dilemma about whether it would be appropriate to include specific counselling on smoking cessation for smokers who attend the clinic. You are not sure if they would take much notice of what you said anyway. You decide to look at the evidence for the effectiveness of advice from nurses on smoking cessation in this primary care setting.

You start by searching on the Cochrane Library. An advanced search on Nurs* AND 'smoking cessation', restricted to the abstract, yields three systematic reviews in the Cochrane Database of Systematic Reviews. One of the abstracts, entitled 'Nursing interventions for smoking cessation' (Rice & Stead 2008), seems relevant to your question. A review of the 'criteria for considering studies' found that studies included were randomised trials in which adult smokers of either gender were recruited in any type of healthcare setting. The types of intervention included the provision of advice, counselling and/or strategies to help patients quit smoking. The main outcome assessed was smoking cessation. The review group divided the interventions into low and high intensity for comparison. A low-intensity intervention was defined as trials where advice was provided during a single consultation lasting up to 10 minutes. A high-intensity intervention was defined as trials where the initial contact lasted more than 10 minutes, with additional materials provided and more than one follow-up session. You were interested to look at the low-intensity comparison separately from the high-intensity comparison, in order to decide which would be the best strategy to implement.

The review included 42 trials. Seven of these evaluated the 'low-intensity' intervention. These results are illustrated in Table 6.6. The pooled relative risk for this group was 1.27 (95% CI 0.99–1.62). As you can see, the combined result indicated by the diamond slightly crosses the vertical line of 'no effect', which means the combined result is not significant. However, the pooled relative risk for the 24 trials of high-intensity interventions, was 1.28 (95% CI 1.18–1.39), are significant. The results for these 24 trials are not shown here, but can be viewed on the Cochrane Library. You were concerned that a number of trials had evaluated nursing interventions for smoking cessation in hospitalised patients and you felt that the results might be better in that setting than in the clinic you were planning to set up. The analysis of all the studies which looked at non-hospitalised patients is shown in Table 6.7. This showed a relative risk of 1.84, indicating a success of well over 50% in the nursing intervention group compared with the control group (RR 1.84, 95% CI 1.49–2.28). Finally, you want to look for evidence of heterogeneity. On examination of the forest plot in Table 6.7 it is clear that the majority of the trials fall to the right-hand side with confidence intervals overlapping. The P-value of 0.32 for the Chi^2 test indicates that no heterogeneity is present. Finally, you are reassured by a value of 12% for the I-squared statistic, again indicating minimal heterogeneity. You conclude that it was appropriate for the 14 trials for non-hospitalised patients to have been pooled in a meta-analysis.

The quality of the review is appraised as described in Box 6.3. The objectives of the review clearly lay out the research question and the right type of study was included.

TABLE 6.6 NURSING INTERVENTIONS FOR SMOKING CESSATION. THE COMPARISON SHOWN IS FOR LOW-INTENSITY INTERVENTION VERSUS CONTROL. THE OUTCOME IS SMOKING CESSATION AT LONGEST FOLLOW-UP (COPYRIGHT COCHRANE LIBRARY, WITH PERMISSION)

Study	Expt n/N	Ctrl n/N	Relative Risk M-H, Fixed, 95% CI	Weight (%)	Relative Risk M-H, Fixed, 95% CI
Low-intensity intervention					
Aveyard 2003	9/413	3/418		0.4	3.04 [0.83, 11.14]
Davies 1992	2/153	4/154		0.5	0.50 [0.09, 2.71]
Janz 1987	26/144	12/106		1.6	1.59 [0.84, 3.01]
Nagle 2005	48/698	54/696		6.4	0.89 [0.61, 1.29]
Nebot 1992	5/81	7/175		0.5	1.54 [0.51, 4.72]
Tonnesen 1996	8/254	3/253		0.4	2.66 [0.71, 9.90]
Vetter 1990	34/237	20/234		2.4	1.68 [1.00, 2.83]
Subtotal (95% CI)	1980	2036		12.1	1.27 [0.99, 1.62]
Total events	132	103			

0.1 0.2　0.5　1　2　5　10
Favours control　　Favours treatment

Heterogeneity: Chi^2 = 9.35, df = 6 (P = 0.16); I^2 = 36%
Test for overall effect: Z = 1.86 (P = 0.063)
Data with permission from Rice et al (2008).

A detailed search strategy has been prepared within the collaborative review group responsible for the review and this is comprehensive. Specific inclusion and exclusion criteria are reported and the quality of the included studies is clearly described. The meta-analysis addressed appropriate comparisons and was easy to understand. The conclusions of the review, which were that 'the results indicate the potential benefits of smoking cessation advice and/or counselling given by nurses to their patients, with reasonable evidence

TABLE 6.7 NURSING INTERVENTIONS FOR SMOKING CESSATION. THE COMPARISON SHOWN IS FOR SMOKING INTERVENTION ALONE VERSUS CONTROL IN NON-HOSPITALISED PATIENTS. THE OUTCOME IS SMOKING CESSATION AT LONGEST FOLLOW-UP (COPYRIGHT COCHRANE LIBRARY, WITH PERMISSION)

Study	Expt n/N	Ctrl n/N	Relative Risk M-H, Fixed, 95% CI	Weight (%)	Relative Risk M-H, Fixed, 95% CI
Smoking intervention alone in other non-hospitalised smokers					
Aveyard 2003	9/413	3/418		2.4	3.04 [0.83,11.14]
Borrelli 2005	9/114	5/120		3.8	1.89 [0.65, 5.48]
Canga 2000	25/147	3/133		2.5	7.54 [2.33, 24.40]
Curry 2003	4/156	3/147		2.4	1.26 [0.29,5.52]
Davies 1992	2/153	4/154		3.1	0.50 [0.09,2.71]
Hilberink 2005	39/244	13/148		12.8	1.82 [1.01, 3.29]
Hollis 1993	79/1997	15/710		17.5	1.87 [1.09,3.23]
Janz 1987	26/144	12/106		10.9	1.59 [0.84,3.01]
Kim 2005	28/200	18/201		14.2	1.56 [0.89,2.73]
Lancaster 1999	8/249	10/248		7.9	0.80 [0.32,1.99]
Nebot 1992	5/81	7/175		3.5	1.54 [0.51,4.72]
Terazawa 2001	8/117	1/111		0.8	7.59 [0.96,59.70]
Tonnesen 1996	8/254	3/253		2.4	2.66 [0.71,9.90]
Vetter 1990	34/237	20/234		15.9	1.68 [1.00,2.83]
Subtotal (95% CI)	4506	3158		100.0	1.84 [1.49,2.28]
Total events	284	117			

0.1 0.2 0.5 1 2 5 10

Favours control   Favours treatment

Heterogeneity: Chi^2 = 14.73, df = 13 (P = 0.32); I^2 = 12%
Test for overall effect: Z = 5.63 (P < 0.00001)

Data with permission from Rice et al (2008).

that the intervention can be effective', appear appropriate and supported by the evidence obtained in the review. You now feel very confident that introducing a smoking cessation strategy (using a high-intensity approach) into your follow-up clinic for patients with risk factors for cardiovascular and respiratory disease will be effective and you are able to go ahead and plan the clinic.

Summary

It will be clear by now that systematic reviews are an important element of evidence-based practice. They are considered the 'gold standard' for assessing the effectiveness of a treatment or intervention. As a research activity, they are important and need to be performed thoroughly. This chapter has described their basic methodology. All practitioners will need to use systematic reviews, so it is important to understand these methods and how the results are presented. They also need to be able to judge the quality of reviews to assess whether their results are valid.

References

CASP checklist, "10 questions to help you make sense of reviews" reproduced with permission from Solutions for Public Health, © *Public Health Resource Unit, England (2006). All rights reserved*, via http://www.phru.nhs.uk/Pages/PHD/resources.htm (accessed 24.06.10).

Cochrane, A.L., 1979. A critical review, with particular reference to the medical profession. In: Teeling-Smith, G. (Ed.), Medicines for the year 2000. Office of Health Economics, London, pp. 1931–1971.

Crowley, P., 1996. Prophylactic corticosteroids for preterm birth (Cochrane Review). Cochrane Database Syst. Rev. (1) Art. No.: CD000065. doi: 10.1002/14651858.CD000065*.

Decullier, E., Lheritier, V., Chapius, F., 2005. Fate of biomedical research protocols and publication bias in France: retrospective cohort study. Br. Med. J. 331, 19.

Decullier, E., Chapuis, F., 2007. Oral presentation bias: a retrospective cohort study. J. Epidemiol. Community Health 61, 190–193.

Easterbrook, P.J., Berlin, J.A., Gopalan, R., Matthews, D.R., 1991. Publication bias in clinical research. Lancet 337, 867–872.

Higgins, J.P.T., Altman, D.G., Sterne, J.A.C (Eds.), Chapter 8: Assessing risk of bias in included studies. In: Higgins, J.P.T, Green, S. (Eds.), Cochrane Handbook for Systematic Reviews of Interventions Version 5.1.0 (updated March 2011). The Cochrane Collaboration, 2011. Avaibale from www.cochrane-handbook.org.

Hooper, L., Harrison, R.A., Summerbell, C.D., et al., 2004. Omega 3 fatty acids for prevention and treatment of cardiovascular disease. Cochrane Database Syst. Rev. 2004 (4) Art. No.: CD003177. doi: 10.1002/14651858.CD003177.pub2*.

Jadad, A.R., Moher, M., Browman, G., Sigouin, C., Fuentes, M., Stevens, R., 2000. Systematic reviews and meta-analyses on treatment of asthma: critical evaluation. Br. Med. J. 320, 537–540.

Kalnins, D., Corey, M., Ellis, L., et al., 2005. Failure of conventional strategies to improve nutritional status in malnourished adolescents and adults with cystic fibrosis. J. Pediatr. 147, 399–401.

Knipschild, P., 1995. Some examples of systematic reviews. In: Chalmers, I., Altman, D.G. (Eds.), Systematic reviews. BMJ Publishing, London, pp. 9–16.

McCarney, R.W., Brinkhaus, B., Lasserson, T.J., Linde, K., 2003. Acupuncture for chronic asthma. Cochrane Database Syst. Rev. 2003 (3) Art. No.: CD000008. doi: 10.1002/14651858. CD000008.pub2*.

McKibbon, A., Hunt, D., Scott Richardson, W., et al., 2005. Finding the evidence. In: Guyatt, G., Rennie, M.D. (Eds.), Users' guides to the medical literature. AMA Press, USA, pp. 21–71.

Nelson, E.A., Prescott, R.J., Harper, D.R., Gibson, B., Brown, D., Ruckley, C.V., 2007. A factorial, randomized trial of pentoxifylline or placebo, four-layer or single-layer compression, and knitted viscose or hydrocolloid dressings for venous ulcers. J. Vasc. Surg. 45 (1), 134–141.

O'Meara, S., Cullum, N.A., Nelson, E.A., 2009. Compression for venous leg ulcers. Cochrane Database Syst. Rev. 2009 (1) Art. No.: CD000265. doi: 10.1002/14651858.CD000265.pub2*.

Pauling, L., 1986. How to live long and feel better. Freeman, New York.

Poustie, V.J., Smyth, R.L., Watling, R.M., 1999. Oral protein calorie supplementation for children with chronic disease. Cochrane Database Syst. Rev. (3) Art. No.: CD001914. doi: 10.1002/14651858.CD001914*.

Rice, V.H., Stead, L.F., 2008. Nursing interventions for smoking cessation. Cochrane Database Syst. Rev. 2008 (1) Art. No.: CD001188. doi: 10.1002/14651858.CD001188.pub3*.

Scherer, R.W., Langenberg, P., von Elm, E., 2007. Full publication of results initially presented in abstracts. Cochrane Database Syst. Rev. (2) Art. No.: MR000005. doi: 10.1002/14651858. MR000005.pub3*.

Schünemann, H.J., Oxman, A.D., Vist, G.E., Higgins, J.P.T., Deeks, J.J., Glasziou, P, Guyatt, G.H. Chapter 12: Interpreting results and drawing conclusions. In: Higgins, J.P.T., Green, S (Eds.), Cochrane Handbook for Systematic Reviews of Interventions Version 5.1.0 (updated March 2011). The Cochrane Collaboration, 2011. Available from www.cochrane-handbook.org.

* Cochrane Reviews are regularly updated as new information becomes available and in response to comments and criticisms. The reader should consult The Cochrane Library for the latest version of a Cochrane Review. Information on The Cochrane Library can be found at http://www.cochrane.org/reviews/clibintro.htm

Further Reading/Internet Resources

Higgins, J.P.T., Green, S. (Eds.), Cochrane Handbook for Systematic Reviews of Interventions Version 5.1.0 [updated March 2011]. The Cochrane Collaboration, 2011. Available from www.cochrane-handbook.org.

Systematic Reviews: CRD's guidance for undertaking reviews in health care 2009. Centre for Reviews and Dissemination 2009. ISBN-978-1900640473.

The Cochrane Collaboration, http://www.cochrane.org/cochrane-reviews.

CHAPTER 7

Evidence-based guidelines

Lois Thomas

KEY POINTS

- There has been an unprecedented increase in guideline development activity in response to professional, public and political calls for evidence-based treatment delivered to comparable standards across the country.

- A potentially unlimited number of clinical topics may be amenable to guideline development. Criteria for topic selection have, therefore, had to be agreed upon.

- Rigorous methods are recommended for guideline development, which is a time-consuming, and often costly, process.

- Guidelines incorporate varying strengths of recommendation according to the strength of the evidence on which they are based.

- Instruments to appraise guidelines should be applied and the quality of the guideline judged before it is accepted for use.
- Strategies for the implementation of guidelines at local and individual clinician level must incorporate methods that have been demonstrated to be effective.

Introduction

Clinical guidelines are 'systematically developed statements to assist practitioner decisions about appropriate health care for specific clinical circumstances' (Field & Lohr 1990). The topic of a clinical guideline may be a condition (such as stroke; Intercollegiate Stroke Working Party 2008) or a symptom (such as incontinence; National Institute for Health and Clinical Excellence (NICE) 2006). For complex conditions, guidelines may be produced to cover different aspects of the disease trajectory; for example, the Canadian Stroke Network/ Heart and Stroke Foundation of Canada and the National Guideline Clearinghouse have produced guidelines on stroke prevention (Lindsay et al 2008a), hyper-acute stroke management (Lindsay et al 2008b), acute inpatient care (Lindsay et al 2008c) and stroke rehabilitation and community integration (Lindsay et al 2008d).

Guidelines can be used to reduce inappropriate variations in practice and to promote the delivery of high-quality, evidence-based health care. They may also provide a mechanism by which healthcare professionals can be made accountable for clinical activities (Falzer et al 2008) and as a basis for regulatory or payer decision-making (American Heart Association 2010). Traditionally, guidelines were based on consensus or individual opinion drawing on personal expertise and/or current practice (and this remains the case in topics or sub-topics where there is little valid research evidence), it is now recognised that guidelines should be explicitly evidence based wherever possible.

To date, most of the development and evaluation of clinical guidelines has been in medicine. The 1990s saw an increase in guidelines in nursing (McClarey 1997, Royal College of Nursing

1995, Von Degenberg & Deighan 1995). The current trend, however, is towards guidelines with a multidisciplinary focus (e.g. Duncan et al 2005) evidenced in the merger of National Collaborating Centres in the UK into one National Clinical Guideline Centre, funded by the NICE and managed by the Royal College of Physicians.

Guideline characteristics

If guidelines are to be effective, it is recommended that they have most, if not all, of the 11 characteristics listed in Table 7.1 (NHS Centre for Reviews and Dissemination (NHS CRD) 1994). Ensuring that guidelines meet these criteria is a resource-intensive task in terms of cost and the time and skills required both in developing evidence-based guidelines and in ensuring they remain up to date. The process from start of guideline development to publication has been estimated by the Scottish Intercollegiate Guidelines Network (SIGN 2008) to take up to 28 months, depending on the volume of relevant literature on the topic, the amount of feedback received during the consultation phase and the time constraints of the guideline development group. The production of a clinical guideline can take up to 2–3 years (Rosenfeld & Shiffman 2009) and cost between £130 000 ($200 000) and £400 000 ($640 000) (Netherlands guidelines and NICE guidelines respectively, Grol 2010). Add to this the complexity of the process and the development of evidence-based guidelines may be beyond the scope of busy practising health professionals.

National or local guideline development

While locally developed ('internal') guidelines may need fewer resources and may be more likely to be adopted into clinical practice because of local ownership (Forrest et al 1996), local groups may not have the extensive skills and resources required for guideline development (Grol 1990). A more common approach is the development of guidelines at regional/national level and subsequent modification to suit local circumstances (Graham & Harrison 2005).

TABLE 7.1 CHARACTERISTICS OF EFFECTIVE GUIDELINES (REPRODUCED FROM NHS CRD 1994 WITH PERMISSION)

Attribute	Explanation
Validity	Evidence should be interpreted correctly so that if a guideline is followed, it leads to the predicted improvements in health
Cost-effectiveness	Improvements in health care should be at acceptable costs. If guidelines ignore issues of costs and concentrate only on benefits, there is the possibility that practices may be recommended with major implications for resource use which are not reflected in correspondingly large improvements in patient outcome
Reproducibility	Given the same evidence, another guideline development group would produce similar recommendations
Reliability	Given the same clinical circumstances another health professional would apply the recommendations in a similar fashion
Representative	All key disciplines and interests contribute to guideline development
Clinical applicability	The target population is defined in accordance with the evidence
Clinical flexibility	Guidelines identify exceptions and indicate how patient preferences are to be incorporated into decision-making
Clarity	Guidelines use precise definitions, unambiguous language and user-friendly formats
Meticulous documentation	Guidelines record participants, assumptions and methods and link recommendations to the available evidence
Scheduled review	Guidelines state when and how they are to be reviewed
Utilisation review	Guidelines indicate ways in which adherence to recommendations can be sensibly monitored

Prioritising topic areas for guideline development

Nationally funded organisations use various criteria to identify the topics that most warrant the significant investments required to develop rigorous evidence-based guidelines. For example, NICE in England endeavours to develop guidance that 'promotes the best possible improvement in public health and wellbeing and/or patient care, and the reduction of inequalities in health, given available resources' (NICE 2008). A selection of questions asked of proposed topics include:

For clinical topics:

• Does the proposed guidance address a condition associated with significant morbidity or mortality in the population as a whole or in particular subgroups?

• Does the proposed guidance focus on interventions or practices that could i) significantly improve patients' or carers' quality of life and/or ii) reduce avoidable morbidity, avoidable premature mortality and/or inequalities in health, relative to current standard practice if the interventions or practices were used more extensively or more appropriately?

Further questions can be found on the NICE website: http://www.nice.org.uk/media/96A/B2/TopicSelectionProcessManualv25.pdf.

In addition, the robustness of the evidence base and whether there is likely to be either inappropriate practice and/or significant variation in clinical practice or access to treatment in the absence of the proposed guideline is considered.

Similarly, SIGN stipulate that there should be a strong research base providing evidence of effective practice to underpin guideline recommendations and that there should be an expectation that change in quality of care and/or patient outcome is possible, desirable and potentially achievable if the guidelines are followed

(SIGN 2008, p18). Additional SIGN criteria for guideline development include:

- Areas of clinical uncertainty as evidenced by wide variation in practice or outcomes.
- Conditions where effective treatment is proven and where mortality or morbidity can be reduced.
- Iatrogenic diseases or interventions carrying significant risks.
- Identified national clinical priority areas: presently these are coronary heart disease and stroke, cancer, and mental health, in addition to improving health and tackling inequalities, especially with regard to children and young people by developing primary and community care and reshaping hospital services.
- The perceived need for the guideline, as indicated by a network of relevant stakeholders.

The idea that guidelines aim to improve quality of care has, at times, been met with scepticism. Some of the earliest criticisms of, or misgivings about, guideline development arose because of cynicism around their purpose; that is, the suspicion that they could be an exercise in cost-containment. Klein (1996) suggests that values, as opposed to research evidence, may determine some judgements made within 'guidelines', citing the example of the accessibility, or limits to the accessibility, of *in vitro* fertilisation treatment (IVF), where value-judgements are made about the ethics of individuals' situations.

In an exercise designed to examine the priorities of nurses in Scotland for the development of 'Best Practice Statements' (www.nhshealthquality.org/nhsqis), which use scientific evidence, where it exists, combined with expert nursing opinion and consensus, topics that topped the poll were nutrition, continence and others that many would consider 'basic' nursing care. Paradoxically, given the treatment costs to the UK National Health Service in these areas, it seems surprising that guideline development groups have not been specifically resourced to develop national guidelines to cover such topics. It may be that a lack of sufficient evidence from randomised controlled trials in these areas has contributed to a dearth of guidelines, but under-researched areas of nursing care, where there may be wide variation in practice, could benefit from being informed by nationally agreed guidelines.

What makes a good guideline? An introduction to the methodology of guideline development

Methods for developing evidence-based guidelines have been formalised at national level, for example in the USA (American Heart Association 2010), Scotland (SIGN 2008), England (NICE 2009), the Netherlands (Dutch Institute for health care improvement, CBO 2006), Australia (the National Health and Medical Research Council (NHMRC) 1999) and New Zealand (the New Zealand Guidelines Group (NZGG) 2003). Recommended stages are presented in Box 7.1.

The guideline development group decides on the scope of the guideline, assesses available research evidence, and produces consensus recommendations which will aid practitioners in their healthcare decisions. According to SIGN (2008), five main skills are required in guideline development group members (but each member is not expected to have the full range):

1. Clinical expertise (e.g. nursing, physiotherapy, etc.)
2. Other specialist expertise (e.g. health economics, research methods)
3. Practical understanding of the problems faced in the delivery of care
4. Communication and team-working skills
5. Critical appraisal skills.

The group should ideally include representatives from all relevant disciplines and interested parties (Lomas 1993a) with representatives seeking the views of their colleagues to ensure that a balanced approach is taken. The optimum size for a group has been put at 8–10 (Scott & Marinker 1990), but groups of between 15 and 25 members have been used successfully (SIGN 2008). A facilitator ensures that all members are free to contribute, that 'decibel level' does not determine priorities (Northern Regional Health

---

BOX 7.1 Stages of guideline development

- Selection of guideline topic
- Composition of the guideline development group
- Defining the scope of the guideline
- Systematic literature review
- Formation of recommendations
- Consultation and peer review
- Presentation and dissemination
- Local implementation
- Audit and review

Authority 1994), and that guideline recommendations accurately reflect the consensus of the whole group.

Involving patients and their relatives in the guideline development process, including identifying questions to underpin reviews of evidence and participation in guideline development groups, is now recommended practice in the UK (e.g. NICE 2009, SIGN 2008); but this may not be the case in other countries. For example, there are few references to patient involvement in the American Heart Association methodology manual (American Heart Association 2010). While anecdotal evidence suggests an active role for patients in guideline development is desirable, there has been very little research into how best to use the patients' expertise in the guideline development process. Furthermore, a recent review found no empirical evidence to support the assumption that active patient participation enhances the quality of clinical guidelines (van de Bovenkamp & Trappenburg 2009). However, patients' knowledge, understanding and experience of their illness means that they are ideally placed to contribute, particularly in areas where guideline development is difficult because of lack of evidence. Involving patients in the process can serve many purposes (SIGN 2008):

- Ensuring guidelines address issues that matter to them
- Highlighting areas where their perspective differs from the views of health professionals
- Reminding other guideline development group members of the limitations of scientific findings in respect of, for example, age, gender, ethnicity, race and quality of life.

While previously patient involvement in guideline development groups was rare (van Wersch & Eccles 1999) and patients who did participate were described as 'non-participating observers' of technical discussions to which their contribution was minimal (Eccles et al 1996), there are now formal structures in place for finding and involving patients at all stages of the process, with clear role definition and support mechanisms (e.g. SIGN 2008). The WHO Advisory Committee on Health Research argue that, while consumers will never comprise representatives from across the spectrum of cultures and settings, their role may be to challenge assumptions about the values used for making guideline recommendations (Schünemann et al 2006a).

Patients involved in guideline development groups have three potential roles; see Table 7.2 for details. In addition it may be beneficial for the advocate (who is not a patient) to have:

- a broad knowledge of the subject of the guideline
- a knowledge of patients' experiences of coping with this symptom or condition
- an awareness of patients' feelings and problems
- an understanding of patients' needs
- training in communication or counselling skills (Van Wersch & Eccles personal communication).

Soliciting patients' views outside the guideline development group and feeding these views back into group discussions may also be effective. This approach was used in the development of the guideline on the recognition and assessment of acute pain in children (Royal College of Nursing 2009): a qualitative study sought children's views and a children's conference was also held, where children described their experiences of

TABLE 7.2 PATIENT ROLES WITHIN GUIDELINE DEVELOPMENT GROUPS

Title	Role
Patient	Presents their own views
Member of patient group	Presents the group's views
Patient advocate	Presents knowledge of patients' views

pain through play, acting, drawing or interview (Doorbar & McClarey 1999).

Once the group has been established, the scope of the guideline is defined (predicated to some extent by available resources), and a number of key clinical questions are identified. A broad topic, for example the management of patients receiving chemotherapy, will take longer to develop and be more labour intensive than a topic that focuses on a single aspect of care such as mouth care in children with cancer.

Next, a detailed literature search is conducted to look for evidence from research studies about the appropriateness and effectiveness of different clinical management strategies. Ideally, this will be evidence from recently updated, rigorously conducted systematic reviews, where appropriate. Further information on systematic reviews is provided in Chapter 6.

Depending on the topic, the search strategy may include only certain study designs. For example, guidelines for the management of hypertension (National Collaborating Centre for Chronic Conditions 2006) only included evidence from randomised controlled trials (RCTs) (ideally these RCTs would be collated within systematic reviews). However, it is common for guideline developers to impose no restriction on study design to answer wider questions than those of effectiveness. The mouth care guideline for children and young people with cancer (CCLG-PONF 2006a) considered the role of health professionals involved in mouth care for the target group, as well as the effectiveness of treatments. The guideline on the recognition and assessment of acute pain in children (Royal College of Nursing 2009) was not concerned with the effectiveness of treatments and included a wider range of study designs.

A level of evidence is allocated to each included publication according to its study design and methodological quality. Studies that have used an appropriate study design to address the research question, and are methodologically sound (for example, for a randomised controlled trial where randomisation, allocation concealment, completeness of follow-up and intention to treat analysis have been adequately performed) are allocated a high level of evidence. Each statement of evidence in the guideline can thus be allocated a level of evidence. For example:

Prostaglandin E is not recommended for the prevention of chemotherapy or radiotherapy induced mucositis as there is evidence that it may promote mucositis. Level B (CCLG-PONF 2006b).

The assigned level indicates the potential for bias within the statement and is taken into consideration when recommendations are formulated. Various scoring systems to assign levels of evidence have been developed, such as GRADE (Atkins et al 2004), adopted by the World Health Organization (Schünemann et al 2006b), and that of SIGN (SIGN 2008), shown in Box 7.2.

BOX 7.2 Statements of evidence

1++	High-quality meta-analyses, systematic reviews of RCTs, or RCTs with a very low risk of bias
1+	Well-conducted meta-analyses, systematic reviews, or RCTs with a low risk of bias
1−	Meta-analyses, systematic reviews, or RCTs with a high risk of bias
2++	High-quality systematic reviews of case control or cohort studies. High-quality case control or cohort studies with a very low risk of confounding or bias and a high probability that the relationship is causal
2+	Well-conducted case control or cohort studies with a low risk of confounding or bias and a moderate probability that the relationship is causal
2−	Case control or cohort studies with a high risk of confounding or bias and a significant risk that the relationship is not causal
3	Non-analytic studies, e.g. case reports, case series
4	Expert opinion

(From SIGN 50, with kind permission of Scottish Intercollegiate Guidelines Network, © Scottish Intercollegiate Guidelines Network (SIGN), 2008.)

Next, the evidence statements (and levels) are considered by the guideline development group and recommendations are formulated. This is a complex part of the process, especially where the evidence can be interpreted in a number of different ways. Methods for translating evidence and professional experiences into recommendations for practice are less sound and transparent than methods used for identifying and grading evidence (Van der Wees et al 2007, Grol 2010). The guideline development group is required to consider all of the evidence relating to each question, in the light of its methodological quality, and make recommendations explicitly based on the most robust evidence. Where recommendations vary, a process for reaching consensus is required. Recommendations are graded according to the level and applicability of evidence to the target population, thus enabling guideline users to assess the predictive validity of each recommendation. An example of grades of recommendation is shown in Box 7.3 (SIGN 2008).

In the absence of high-quality research evidence to underpin all or some guideline recommendations, the views of a group of experts may be distilled through a consensus development process (Fink et al 1984). Using this process enables guidelines to cover all the areas where clinicians need to make decisions rather than restricting the guideline scope to researched areas only. Useful pointers for the process of consensus development of guidelines are provided by Murphy et al. (1998). A recent synthesis of systematic review findings examining the effectiveness of clinical guideline implementation strategies found that guidelines produced by consensus methods or by end-users increased clinical ownership and led to up to 40% improvements in compliance or desired practice (Prior et al 2008).

Achieving consensus is not easy and may be hampered by the most assertive or most authoritative group members having a greater say than others (Thomson et al 1995). There are, however, ways of getting the best out of a group, such as the Delphi technique or the nominal group technique (Jones & Hunter 1995), although Murphy et al (1998) sound a note of caution

---

BOX 7.3 Grades of recommendation

A
At least one meta analysis, systematic review, or RCT rated as 1++, and directly applicable to the target population; or
A body of evidence consisting principally of studies rated as 1+, directly applicable to the target population, and demonstrating overall consistency of results

B
A body of evidence including studies rated as 2++, directly applicable to the target population, and demonstrating overall consistency of results; or
Extrapolated evidence from studies rated as 1++ or 1+

C
A body of evidence including studies rated as 2+, directly applicable to the target population and demonstrating overall consistency of results; or
Extrapolated evidence from studies rated as 2++

D
Evidence level 3 or 4; or
Extrapolated evidence from studies rated as 2+

GOOD PRACTICE POINTS
☑ Recommended best practice based on the clinical experience of the guideline development group.

(From SIGN 50, with kind permission of Scottish Intercollegiate Guidelines Network, © Scottish Intercollegiate Guidelines Network (SIGN), 2008.)

---

suggesting that, while using the Delphi or nominal group technique may result in convergence of individual judgements, it is not clear whether the accuracy of the group decision is increased.

The Delphi technique does not require group members to meet; instead group members generate topics of discussion. These are sent to all participants, who then comment, in writing, on their co-participants' views. Responses are analysed and collated and sent back to participants. The process continues until a consensus is reached.

A modified Delphi style approach was used in the **Mouth Care for Children and Young People with Cancer guideline** (Glenny et al. 2010, CCLG-PONF 2006a) to develop recommendations in dental care and basic oral hygiene, as there was little evidence in these particular areas. Statements were drawn up by the guideline development team, based on the opinions of team members, and a survey of current oral care practice conducted in UK children's cancer care centres. These were circulated to members of the cancer care centres, the Paediatric Oncology Nurses Forum, paediatric dentists and dental hygienists, and respondents were asked to grade each statement from 1 (strongly disagree) to 5 (strongly agree). Responses were used to construct provisional recommendations, which were then subject to peer review.

The nominal group technique achieves consensus using highly structured meetings. In brief, it comprises two rounds in which participants write down their views on the topic then offer them up, in turn, to be recorded on a flip chart. Suggestions are discussed then privately rated by each member; ratings are tabulated, discussed and re-rated. The method can also be used within a single meeting and, in the context of guideline development, includes a detailed review of the literature as background material for the topic under discussion. A modified version of the nominal group technique was used in the development of the pressure ulcer risk assessment and prevention guideline (Rycroft-Malone & McInness 2000). The process is outlined in Table 7.3.

Guideline recommendations should be written in 'plain English', which means avoiding highly technical language and using active rather than passive verbs, and appropriate numerical information should be included. The use of this approach has been linked with stronger intentions to implement the guidelines and more positive attitudes towards them (Michie & Lester 2005).

Finally, the guideline is tested by asking professionals not involved in guideline development to review it for clarity, internal consistency and acceptability. The guideline can be piloted in selected healthcare settings to see whether its use is feasible in routine practice.

TABLE 7.3 MODIFIED NOMINAL GROUP TECHNIQUE USED TO DEVELOP THE PRESSURE ULCER RISK ASSESSMENT AND PREVENTION GUIDELINE (RYCROFT-MALONE & MCINNESS 2000, REPRODUCED WITH PERMISSION FROM THE ROYAL COLLEGE OF NURSING)

Stage	Process
Formation of consensus group	A group of 10 people reflecting the full range of people to which the guideline will apply was formed using purposive sampling based on the parameters of status, knowledge of the research and intended commitment to the process.
Synthesis of pertinent information	Consensus group provided with relevant research and two systematic reviews.
Ranking of statements	Before the group meeting, participants asked to consider 200 statements developed from the literature and evidence-linked recommendations. Each participant was asked to rate agreement on each statement on a scale of 1–9 (1, least agreement; 9, most agreement). Frequency of response to each statement calculated. Pattern of responses for the group presented alongside each members' response to each statement.
Nominal group meeting	Statements discussed in turn, focusing primarily on those where there was most disagreement. All members given chance to respond; followed by discussion to clarify, defend or dispute issues. Participants given the opportunity to privately re-rate statements.
Mathematical aggregation	Median (measurement of central tendency or average) and inter-quartile range (measure of distribution) calculated from each statement from ratings of second round. Statements with a median of 7–9 developed into practice recommendations.
Development of recommendations	Recommendations drafted based on panel's level of agreement about the statements.

All guidelines should be reviewed after a specified time period to make sure they are updated to take into account new knowledge. Frequency of review will depend on the amount of new information in the particular topic area. If there have been significant developments in the evidence base, review may need to take place to incorporate these.

Example of an evidence-based guideline

The guideline for *Mouth Care for Children and Young People with Cancer* (Glenny et al. 2010, CCLG-PONF 2006a) was produced in 2006 and, as described above, contains both 'best practice' (based on consensus indicated by √) and evidence-based recommendations that are graded using the SIGN grading system. An example showing a range of recommendations is given in Box 7.4.

Appraising published guidelines

Developing new evidence-based guidelines is expensive and time-consuming and it is, therefore, preferable, in the majority of cases, to seek out previously published guidelines if these are locally applicable and of good quality. Some useful websites for finding guidelines are given at the end of this chapter. A validated instrument used internationally is available for appraising the quality of published guidelines (AGREE 2001). An exercise in guideline appraisal using the mouth care for children and young people with cancer guideline (Glenny et al. 2010, CCLG-PONF 2006a) is available on the website.

While using this tool will give a good indication of guideline quality, it is likely that many will not score highly on all sections of the instrument. A recent evaluation of seven guidelines on depression showed scores of 25–63% for stakeholder involvement, 1–64% for rigour of development, 0–56% for applicability and 8–75% for editorial independence (Hegarty et al 2009).

BOX 7.4 Example of recommendations

Recommendations for the prevention of oral mucositis

Parents and patients should be informed of the   Grade √
importance of keeping the mouth clean and
encouraged to practise good, basic oral hygiene.

The following have all been shown to be potentially beneficial   Grade B
for the prevention of mucositis in adult populations. Their
use in children for the prevention of radiotherapy- and/or
chemotherapy-induced mucositis can only be considered
within the constraints of an RCT: amifostine, allopurinol
mouthwash (for 5-FU therapy), ice-chips, GM-CSF/GCSF,
benzydamine, antibiotic pastilles/pastes (containing PTA),
povidine-iodine, pilocarpine (not currently available in a form
suitable for children), hydrolitic enzymes.

RCTs of allupurinol mouthwash are not recommended   Grade D
for children receiving cancer treatment other than 5-FU.

Prostaglandin E is not recommended for the prevention   Grade B
of chemotherapy- or radiotherapy-induced mucositis as
there is evidence that it may promote mucositis.

(From the Glenny et al 2010 Mouth Care for Children and Young People with Cancer
guideline, with permission)

Adapting nationally developed guidelines for local use

The translation of nationally developed or other guidelines developed 'externally' into protocols for local use is both permissible and, in the opinion of many commentators, desirable. Feder et al (1999) suggest that, just as topics for guideline development require to be prioritised against a set of accepted criteria, so local organisations must develop a system for prioritising the implementation of guidelines locally. The sheer volume of recommendations contained within all of the clinical guidelines that might be applicable to the work of a general practitioner, for example make prioritising according to local need a necessity.

Local adaptation of guidelines also has the potential for mitigating some of the objections to their use detailed below; for example, that they may lack local relevance. Asking local clinical teams to appraise 'external' guidelines and prioritise their implementation may also bring a sense of ownership that can be difficult to achieve otherwise.

Issues of resource availability and potential returns, in terms of health gain, also need to be considered. This, though, raises the issue of when local adaptation becomes unacceptable, potentially recreating the situation guidelines are designed to address. NICE has issued guidance on the use of beta-interferon for people with multiple sclerosis and has made a judgement against its use (NICE 2002; decision upheld in 2007). Had they decided for its use, it may have had little effect on the budgets of some Health Authorities/Boards in areas of low incidence, whilst in other areas where there is a higher than average incidence of multiple sclerosis (as in the South West of Scotland in the UK), the costs would have been high and would arguably have meant that other services could have suffered as a result.

Patient versions of guidelines

Versions of guidelines that are accessible to and are written for patients, often in a range of languages, are now common practice. For example, in the USA many guidelines found in the Agency for Healthcare Research and Quality National Guideline Clearinghouse have a 'patient resources' section compiled by the guideline developer, as well as links to many relevant websites; NICE produces all its guidelines in formats accessible to patients, carers and the public; there are patient versions available of the Inter-collegiate National Clinical Guidelines on Stroke (Intercollegiate Working Party for Stroke 2008 http://www.rcplondon.ac.uk/pubs/contents/a8bf7a9f-a150-4727-8a96-3f09e6175ce5.pdf). There has, however, been little research into the impact of guidelines in helping patients manage their condition.

Introducing the guideline into practice

Once a clinical guideline is ready for use, two stages facilitate its introduction into practice: dissemination and implementation. Dissemination is generally taken to refer to the method by which the guidelines are made available to potential users. Strategies include publication in professional journals, sending the guideline to targeted individuals and educational interventions. Several studies have assessed the effectiveness of such strategies: dissemination by publication or direct mailing have been found to have a beneficial effect on process outcomes, but not patient outcomes (Farmer et al 2008), and have the advantage of being cheap and reproducible. Strategies involving an educational component, especially where this is specifically targeted rather than in the form of continuing education, are more likely to result in behaviour change: educational outreach visits (O'Brien et al 2007), and continuing education meetings and workshops (Forsetlund et al 2009) have also been shown to have a small effect. However, dissemination alone without an appropriate implementation strategy is unlikely to influence behaviour significantly (Grimshaw et al 1995).

Implementation is a means of ensuring that users subsequently act upon the recommendations. 'Implementation is a more active process, involving tailoring the message to the needs of the target audience, and actively working to overcome barriers to behaviour change' (Lomas 1993b). Implementation strategies try to ensure that users adopt and apply guidelines to which they have access. Using a range of intervention strategies has been found to lead consistently to significant improvements in guideline compliance and behaviour change (Prior et al 2008) and to show greater evidence of effectiveness than using single interventions. The number of components needed to increase effectiveness and the effect of combining different strategies is, however, not yet known. Grol (1992) recommends that implementation plans take account of barriers to behaviour change; these may include both structural and attitudinal factors. A group in Australia is developing a tool to identify potential problems in implementing guideline recommendations, the

GuideLine Implementability Appraisal (GLIA) tool, for use by guideline developers to refine guidelines during their development phase (Hill & Lalor 2010).

Some implementation strategies supply accessible reminders of the guideline and decision support systems (often computer based). These have been shown to lead to significant practice improvements (Prior et al 2008). A recent realistic evaluation of protocol-based care found protocols were referred to more often when they were physically close to the patient-practitioner interaction and/or easily accessible, e.g. onscreen (Rycroft-Malone et al 2010). Audit and feedback has also been shown to be capable of affecting professional behaviour: a systematic review of randomised controlled trials found audit and feedback can be effective in improving professional practice and healthcare outcomes, with effects generally small to moderate (Jamtvedt et al 2006). The Cochrane review of local opinion leaders (people viewed as being likeable, trustworthy and influential; Doumit et al 2007) has also concluded that their use can successfully promote evidence-based practice.

The involvement of patients in dissemination and implementation requires further attention, but could potentially serve to enhance the use of guidelines in practice (Burgers et al 2003).

A systematic review of the effectiveness and efficiency of guideline dissemination and implementation strategies targeting medically qualified healthcare professionals (Grimshaw et al 2004) found all interventions achieved improvements in care. A median absolute improvement in performance of 14.1% was found in cluster randomised comparisons of reminders, 8.1% in cluster randomised comparisons of dissemination of educational materials, 7.0% in cluster randomised comparisons of audit and feedback and 6.0% in cluster randomised comparisons of multifaceted interventions involving educational outreach. Only one-quarter of studies included economic data on the costs of developing guidelines and introducing them into practice. Healthcare organisations, therefore, have little evidence to inform decisions on whether the costs involved in guideline development and introduction do not outweigh potential benefits.

There are few studies evaluating dissemination and implementation strategies in nursing (Richens et al 2004). The systematic review by Thomas et al (1999) found three studies evaluating dissemination and implementation strategies; findings appear to suggest that educational interventions (e.g. lectures, teaching sessions) are of more value than passive approaches (e.g. postal distribution) in the dissemination of guidelines. However, methodological flaws limit the credibility of findings. Further research is needed into the roles nurses and other professions play in guideline dissemination and implementation, as what is effective for doctors may not be for nurses (Richens et al 2004, Puffer & Rashidian 2004).

Evaluating the effectiveness of clinical guidelines in nursing and allied health professions

Most of the literature on clinical guidelines comes from medicine. However, a systematic review for the Cochrane Collaboration examined whether clinical guidelines are effective in changing the behaviour of nurses, midwives and health visitors and other allied health professions (Thomas et al 1999). Eighteen evaluations of guidelines were found; all but one of these studies evaluated the introduction of guidelines targeting nurses. Key findings of the systematic review are summarized in Box 7.5, but interested readers are encouraged to keep an eye out for the next update to the systematic review, being undertaken by Harrison et al, due for publication on the Cochrane Database of Systematic Reviews (http://www.thecochranelibrary.com).

Whilst this review has provided some evidence that guideline-driven care can be effective in changing the practice of nurses and patient outcomes, there is a long way to go before guidelines meeting the eleven criteria (Table 7.1) are routinely used by nurses to improve patient care. The trend towards centralisation of guideline development and the production of guidelines designed to be used by the multidisciplinary team, including nurses, has led to a wide repertoire of high-quality guidelines. The focus is now

> **BOX 7.5** Key points from systematic review of the effectiveness of clinical guidelines in nursing, midwifery and professions allied to medicine (Thomas et al 1999)
>
> - Significant changes in some processes of care were found in four out of five studies measuring process.
> - Six out of eight studies measuring outcomes found significant differences favouring the group who received guidelines.
> - Three studies evaluated dissemination and implementation strategies: findings appear to suggest that educational interventions (e.g. lectures, teaching sessions) are of more value than passive approaches (e.g. postal distribution) in the dissemination of guidelines; however, methodological flaws limit the credibility of findings.
> - Studies examining the ability of guidelines to enable skill substitution generally support the hypothesis of no difference between nurse protocol-driven and physician care.

shifting to 'implementation research' in order to understand what promotes the introduction of guidelines into practice, in what circumstances, and why (Middleton et al 2009).

Benefits and disbenefits of clinical guidelines

Clinical guidelines, integrated care pathways, protocols of care and any other externally imposed directives pertaining to the treatment of and interventions used on patients (i.e. any directive about a clinician's action which individual clinicians may not have been involved in devising) will arguably all face the same set of objections, misconceptions and concerns about their use and, importantly, their legal standing. Hurwitz (1999) points out that 'Courts are unlikely to adopt standards of care advocated in clinical guidelines as legal "gold standards" because the mere fact that the guideline exists does not of itself establish that compliance with it is reasonable in the circumstances, or that non-compliance is negligent'. He also states that guidelines should not be viewed as 'thought-proof', but that they require interpretation and the use of discretion. SIGN (2008) and NICE (2009) suggest that significant deviations from the guideline, together with reasons for these, are documented in patients' case notes at the time the decision is taken.

Objections to, and support for, the use of guidelines are based on differing perceptions of the problems they are designed to address and of the related benefits or disbenefits they bring.

The use of guidelines has been criticised on the grounds that they can:

- stifle individual clinical judgement
- de-skill professionals by reducing their capacity to think for themselves
- limit quality of care by restricting care/treatment options
- introduce practice which could be ineffective or dangerous
- encourage the illusion that there is clear-cut direction to be taken in every clinical situation
- be resource-intensive in development and implementation
- lack local relevance
- concentrate on 'easy' areas, that is where there is already a body of evidence about appropriate treatment
- allow powerful and vocal individuals to impose their priorities on particular services
- require clinicians to follow courses of action for which they do not have the requisite skills or knowledge
- raise patient expectations about types and standards of care they might expect to receive.

For each of these criticisms or objections there is an opposing assertion or opinion. It has been suggested that guidelines:

- ensure safe practice
- improve consistency of care in different parts of the country/ settings of care
- make it more likely that patients receive correct treatment

- build parity of knowledge amongst staff
- bring expert opinion to everyday clinical care
- allow for individual patient variation – non-application is not disallowed, but requires justification
- provide more information for patients about what they should expect from the healthcare system
- distill the vast array of knowledge relating to individual clinical conditions into a manageable guide for busy clinicians
- allow room for the development of local protocols.

The restriction of individual clinical judgement and the apparent requirement to treat all patients the same, regardless of individual idiosyncrasies or characteristics, seems to be at the heart of most objections to or difficulties with the use of guidelines. Likewise the heart of the defence case for the use of guidelines seems to be the argument that patients deserve the best possible treatment all of the time in definable situations regardless of the individual expertise of the person dealing with them at the time; if guidelines can expedite that best treatment, the argument goes, then they have a legitimate place in the system.

The acid test for clinical guidelines and the answer to any criticisms would surely proceed from proof of their benefit to patient care. As outlined above, more studies are needed to assess the impact of guidelines, particularly in nursing and allied health professions.

Conclusion

If guidelines are to be underpinned by evidence of effective practice, a prerequisite is high-quality evidence of the benefits, harms and costs of the procedures and practices targeted and, just as importantly, of patients' needs and preferences. Further research into is required to provide this evidence base.

Nurses whose behaviour is targeted by guidelines need to have an active role in their development or adaptation to local circumstances: this approach will encourage 'ownership' of the guideline and is more likely to lead to more positive attitudes towards it. It will also ensure that profession-specific practices and barriers, and any factors that facilitate behaviour change, are taken into account.

Where possible, the introduction of clinical guidelines should be within an evaluative framework to help build evidence of effective implementation strategies.

Clinical guidelines are a potential means by which evidence can be incorporated into nursing practice. However, more research is clearly required to underpin clinical recommendations and to assess the most effective ways of developing, disseminating and implementing clinical guidelines in nursing. Only then will a decision be possible about their potential for improving nursing practice and patient outcomes.

References

AGREE, 2001. Appraisal of Guidelines Research and Evaluation Instrument. Health Care Evaluation Unit at St George's Hospital Medical School, London. www.agreecollaboration.org.

American Heart Association, 2010. Methodology manual for ACCF/AHA guideline writing committees. www.americanheart.org/presenter.jhtml?identifier=3039684 (accessed 1st July 2010).

Atkins, D., Best, D., Briss, P.A., et al., 2004. Grading quality of evidence and strength of recommendations. Br. Med. J. 328 (7454), 1490.

Burgers, J.S., Grol, R., Klazinga, N.S., Mäkelä, M., Zaat, J. for the AGREE Collaboration, 2003. Towards evidence-based clinical practice: an international survey of 18 clinical guideline programs. Int. J. Qual. Health Care 15 (1), 31–45.

CBO, 2006. Evidence-based richtlijnontwikkeling. Handleiding voor werkgroepleden. Kwaliteitsintituut voor de gezondheitszorg CBO, Utrecht. http://www.cbo.nl.

CCLG-PONF Mouth Care Group, 2006a. Mouth care for children and young people with cancer: evidence-based guidelines. Guideline Report. http://www.cclg.org.uk/treatmentandresearch/content.php?2id=19.

CCLG-PONF Mouth Care Group, 2006b. Mouth care for children and young people with cancer: evidence-based guidelines. Methodological Report. http://www.cclg.org.uk/treatmentandresearch/content.php?2id=19.

Doorbar, P., McClarey, M., 1999. Ouch! sort it out: children's experiences of pain. RCN Publishing, London.

Doumit, G., Gattellari, M., Grimshaw, J., O'Brien, M.A., 2007. Local opinion leaders: effects on professional practice and health care outcomes. Cochrane Database Syst Rev (1). Art. No.:CD000125. doi:10.1002/14651858.CD000125.pub3.

Duncan, P.W., Zorowitz, R., Bates, B., et al., 2005. Management of adult stroke rehabilitation care: a clinical practice guideline. Stroke 36, 100–143.

Eccles, M.P., Clapp, Z., Grimshaw, J., et al., 1996. Developing valid guidelines: methodological and procedural issues from the North of England evidence based guideline development project. Qual. Health Care 5, 44–50.

Falzer, P.R., Moore, B.A., Garman, D.M., 2008. Incorporating clinical guidelines through clinician decision-making. Implementation Science 3, 13.

Farmer, A.P., Légaré, F., Turcot, L., Grimshaw, J., Harvey, E., McGowan, J.L., et al., 2008. Printed educational materials: effects on professional practice and health care outcomes. Cochrane Database Syst. Rev. (3). Art. No.:CD004398. doi:10.1002/14651858.CD004398.pub2.

Feder, G., Eccles, M., Grol, R., Griffiths, C., Grimshaw, J., 1999. Using clinical guidelines. Br. Med. J. 318 (7185), 728–730.

Field, M.J., Lohr, K.N., 1990. Clinical practice guidelines: directions for a new program. National Academy Press, Washington, DC.

Fink, A., Kosecoff, J., Chassin, M., Brook, R.H., 1984. Consensus methods: characteristics and guidelines for use. Am. J. Public Health 74 (9), 979–983.

Forrest, D., Hoskins, A., Hussey, R., 1996. Clinical practice guidelines and their implementation. Postgrad. Med. 72, 19–22.

Forsetlund, L., Bjørndal, A., Rashidian, A., Jamtvedt, G., O'Brien, M.A., Wolf, F., et al., 2009. Continuing education meetings and workshops: effects on professional practice and health care outcomes. Cochrane Database Syst. Rev. (2). Art.No.:CD003030. doi:10.1002/14651858.CD003030.pub2.

Glenny, A.M., Gibson, F., Auld, E., et al., on behalf of the Children's Cancer and Leukaemia Group/Paediatric Oncology Nurses Forum's (CCLG/PONF) Mouth Care Group, 2010. The development of evidence-based guidelines on mouth care for children, teenagers and young adults treated for cancer. Eur. J. Cancer 46, 1399–1412.

Graham, I.D., Harrison, M., 2005. Evaluation and adaptation of clinical practice guidelines. Evid. Based Nurs. 8, 68–72.

Grimshaw, J., Freemantle, N., Wallace, S., et al., 1995. Developing and implementing clinical practice guidelines. Qual. Health Care 4, 55–64.

Grimshaw, J.M., Thomas, R.E., MacLennan, G., et al., 2004. Effectiveness and efficiency of guideline dissemination and implementation strategies. Health Technol. Assess. 8 (6), iii–iiv, 1–72.

Grol, R., 1990. National standard setting for quality of care in general practice: attitudes of general practitioners and response to a set of standards. Br. J. Gen. Pract. 40, 361–364.

Grol, R., 1992. Implementing guidelines in general practice care. Qual. Health Care 1 (3), 184–191.

Grol, R., 2010. Has guideline development gone astray? Yes. Br. Med. J. 340, c306.

Hegarty, K., Gunn, J., Blashki, G., Griffith, T., Dowell, T., Kendrick, T., 2009. How could depression guidelines be made more relevant and applicable to primary care? Br. J. Gen. Pract. 59, 322–328.

Hill, K.M., Lalor, E.E., 2010. How useful is an online tool to facilitate guideline implementation? Feasibility study of using eGLIA by stroke clinicians in Australia. Qual. Saf. Health Care 18, 157–159.

Hurwitz, B., 1999. Legal and political considerations of clinical practice guidelines. Br. Med. J. 318 (7184), 661–664.

Intercollegiate Stroke Working Party, 2008. National clinical guidelines for stroke, third ed. RCP, London.

Intercollegiate Working Party for Stroke, 2008. Care after stroke: information for patients and their carers. Royal College of Physicians, London.

Jamtvedt, G., Young, J.M., Kristoffersen, D.T., O'Brien, M.A., Oxman, A.D., 2006. Audit and feedback: effects on professional practice and health care outcomes. Cochrane Database Syst. Rev. (2). Art.No.:CD000259. doi:10.1002/14651858.CD000259.pub2.

Jones, J., Hunter, D., 1995. Consensus methods for medical and health services research. Br. Med. J. 311, 376–380.

Klein, R., 1996. The NHS and the new scientism: solution or delusion? Q. J. Med. 89, 85–87.

Lindsay, P., Bayley, M., Hellings, C., Hill, M., Woodbury, E., Phillips, S., 2008a. Prevention of stroke. Blood pressure management. In: Canadian best practice recommendations for stroke care Can. Med. Assoc. J. 179 (Suppl. 12), E19–E22.

Lindsay, P., Bayley, M., Hellings, C., Hill, M., Woodbury, E., Phillips, S., 2008b. Hyperacute stroke management. Emergency medical services management of acute stroke patients. In: Canadian best practice recommendations for stroke care. Can. Med. Assoc. J. 179 (Suppl. 12), E33–E35.

Lindsay, P., Bayley, M., Hellings, C., Hill, M., Woodbury, E., Phillips, S., 2008c. Acute inpatient stoke care. Stroke unit care. In: Canadian best practice recommendations for stroke care. Can. Med. Assoc. J. 179 (Suppl. 12), E45–E48.

Lindsay, P., Bayley, M., Hellings, C., Hill, M., Woodbury, E., Phillips, S., 2008d. Stroke rehabilitation and community reintegration. Provision of inpatient stroke rehabilitation. In: Canadian best practice recommendations for stroke care. Can. Med. Assoc. J. 179 (Suppl. 12), E54–E56.

Lomas, J., 1993a. Making clinical policy explicit. Legislative policy making and lessons for developing practice guidelines. Int. J. Technol. Assess. Health Care 9, 11–25.

Lomas, J., 1993b. Teaching old (and not so old) docs new tricks: effective ways to implement research findings. Working paper 93–4. McMaster University Centre for Health Economics and Policy Analysis, Toronto.

McClarey, M., 1997. Identifying priorities for guideline development as a result of nursing needs. DQI Network News 6, 4–5.

Michie, S., Lester, K., 2005. Words matter: increasing the implementation of clinical guidelines. Qual. Saf. Health Care 14, 367–370.

Middleton, S., Levi, C., Ward, J., et al., 2009. Fever, hyperglycaemia and swallowing dysfunction management in acute stroke: a cluster randomized controlled trial of knowledge transfer. Implementation Science 4, 16.

Murphy, M.K., Black, N.A., Lamping, D.L., et al., 1998. Consensus development methods and their use in clinical guideline development. Health Technol. Assess. 2 (3), i–iv, 1–88.

National Collaborating Centre for Chronic Conditions, 2006. Hypertension: management in adults in primary care: pharmacological update. Royal College of Physicians, London.

National Institute for Health and Cinical Excellence, 2002. Beta interferon and glatiramer acetate for the treatment of multiple schlerosis. National Institute for Health and Clinical Excellence, London.

National Institute for Health and Clinical Excellence, 2006. Urinary incontinence: The management of urinary incontinence in women. NICE Clinical Guideline, 40. National Institute for Health and Clinical Excellence, London.

National Institute for Health and Clinical Excellence, 2008. Topic Selection Programme Process Manual. http://www.nice.org.uk/media/96A/B2/TopicSelectionProcessManualv25.pdf.

National Institute for Health and Clinical Excellence, 2009. The Guideline Development Process. National Institute for Clinical Excellence, London. www.nice.org.uk.

NHMRC, 1999. A guide to the development, implementation and evaluation of clinical practice guidelines. National Health and Medical Research Council (NHMRC), Canberra. http://www.nhmrc.gov.au.

NHS Centre for Reviews and Dissemination, 1994. Implementing clinical practice guidelines. University of Leeds, Leeds.

Northern Regional Health Authority, 1994. Guidelines – a resource pack. Northern Regional Health Authority, Newcastle upon Tyne, pp. 1–40.

NZGG, 2003. Handbook for the preparation of explicit evidence-based clinical practice guidelines. New Zealand Guidelines Group, Wellington. http://www.nzgg.org.nz.

O'Brien, M.A., Rogers, S., Jamtvedt, G., et al., 2007. Educational outreach visits: effects on professional practice and health care outcomes. Cochrane Database Syst. Rev. (4). Art.No.:CD000409. doi:10.1002/14651858.CD000409.pub2.

Prior, M., Guerin, M., Grimmer-Somers, 2008. The effectiveness of clinical guideline implementation strategies – a synthesis of systematic review findings. J. Eval. Clin. Pract. 14, 888–897.

Puffer, S., Rashidian, A., 2004. Practice nurses' intentions to use clinical guidelines. J. Adv. Nurs. 47 (5), 500–509.

Richens, Y., Anderson, E.G., Rycroft-Malone, J., Morrell, C., 2004. Getting guidelines into practice: a literature review. Nurs. Stand. 18, 33–40.

Rosenfeld, R.M., Shiffman, R.N., 2009. Clinical practice guideline development manual: a quality-driven approach for translating evidence into action. Otolaryngol. Head Neck Surg. 140 (6 Suppl. 1), S1–S43.

Royal College of Nursing, 1995. Clinical guidelines: what you need to know. Royal College of Nursing, London.

Royal College of Nursing, 2009. The recognition and assessment of acute pain in children. Royal College of Nursing, London.

Rycroft-Malone, J., McInness, E., 2000. Pressure ulcer risk assessment and prevention. Technical Report Royal College of Nursing, London.

Rycroft-Malone, J., Fontenla, M., Bick, D., Seers, K., 2010. A realistic evaluation: the case of protocol-based care. Implementation Science 5, 38.

Schünemann, H.J., Fretheim, A., Oxman, A.D., 2006a. Improving the use of research evidence in guideline development: 10. Integrating values and consumer involvement. Health Research Policy and Systems 4, 22.

Schünemann, H.J., Fretheim, A., Oxman, A.D., 2006b. Improving the use of research evidence in guideline development: 9. Grading evidence and recommendations. Health Research Policy and Systems 4, 21.

Scott, M., Marinker, M.L., 1990. Medical audit and general practice. Br. Med. J. London.

SIGN (Scottish Intercollegiate Guidelines Network), 2008. A guideline developers' handbook, Revised ed. SIGN publication no. 50. http://www.sign.ac.uk/guidelines/fulltext/50/.

Thomas, L.H., Cullum, N.A., McColl, E., Rousseau, N., Soutter, J., Steen, N., 1999. Guidelines in professions allied to medicine.

Cochrane Database Syst. Rev. (1). Art.No.:CD000349. doi:10.1002/14651858.CD000349.

Thomson, R., Lavender, M., Madhok, R., 1995. How to ensure that guidelines are effective. Br. Med. J. 311, 237–242.

van de Bovenkamp, H.M., Trappenburg, M.J., 2009. Reconsidering patient participation in guideline development. Health Care Anal. 17, 198–216.

Van der Wees, P.J., Hendriks, E.J.M., Custers, J.W.H., Burgers, J.S., Dekker, J., de Bie, R.A., 2007. Comparison of international guideline programs to evaluate and update the Dutch program for clinical guideline development in physical therapy. BMC Health Serv. Res. 7, 191.

Van Wersch, A., Eccles, M., 1999. Patient involvement in evidence-based health in relation to clinical guidelines. In: Gabbay, M. (Ed.), The evidence-based primary care handbook. Royal Society of Medicine Press, London, pp. 91–103.

Von Degenberg, K., Deighan, M., 1995. Guideline development: A model of multi-professional collaboration. In: Deighan, M., Hitch, S. (Eds.), Clinical effectiveness from guidelines to cost-effective practice. Department of Health, London, pp. 93–97.

APPENDIX 7.1

Useful Websites

Agency for Healthcare Research and Quality

www.ahrq.gov

Canadian Medical Association

http://www.gacguidelines.ca/

eGUIDELINES

http://www.eguidelines.co.uk/

Guidelines International Network

http://www.g-i-n.net/

National Clinical Guideline Centre

http://www.ncgc.ac.uk/

National Electronic Library for Health guidelines database

http://www.nelh.nhs.uk/guidelines_database.asp

National Guideline Clearinghouse

http://www.guideline.gov

New Zealand Guidelines Group

http://www.nzgg.org.nz/index.cfm

National Health and Medical Research Council

http://www7.health.gov.au/nhmrc/publications/index.htm

National Institute for Health and Clinical Excellence

http://www.nice.org.uk/

National Library of Medicine (available via PubMed)

http://www.ncbi.nlm.nih.gov/pubmed

The Royal College of Nursing (RCN clinical guidelines can be accessed from this site)

http://www.rcn.org.uk/development/practice/clinicalguidelines

Scottish Intercollegiate Guidelines Network

http://www.show.scot.nhs.uk/sign/guidelines/

CHAPTER

Using research evidence in making clinical decisions with individual patients

Dawn Dowding and Carl Thompson

KEY POINTS

- Evidence from high-quality research studies should form the basis for making clinical decisions with and for individual patients.
- Techniques such as Bayesian probability revision and decision analysis are useful tools to assist with making clinical decisions for individual patients.
- An evidence-based decision should incorporate patient values and their preferences for different treatments or outcomes.

- Be aware that how we communicate information to patients can affect the decisions they take.
- How individuals understand risks and benefits differs. Consider communicating the same information in different ways.
- Decision support tools and decision aids can help incorporate evidence into clinical decisions.

Introduction

The terms 'clinical judgement' (Benner & Tanner 1987, Itano 1989), 'clinical reasoning' (Grobe et al 1991), and 'clinical decision making' (Field 1987) all describe the same phenomenon: using information to make judgements (evaluations) and decisions (choices) about a patient's condition. In an evidence-based approach to patient care, the information should be the highest quality research evidence we can access. However, research evidence is not the only component of evidence-based decisions; a patient's preferences for different treatments or outcomes and the availability (or lack thereof) of funds, resources and clinical skill/expertise to provide a particular intervention are also important components in the decision process (DiCenso et al 1998). Furthermore, making clinical decisions with individual patients involves not just considering the implications of the evidence for that patient, but also helping them to apply it to their own individual circumstances.

One of the challenges of evidence-based practice is that of knowing how to take the research evidence generated by studying samples of patients and apply it to the decisions made with individual patients. In this chapter, we examine practical ways in which you can do this and discuss approaches that you can use to help patients to understand the evidence, so assisting them with their decision-making. We consider how you can take into account patients' views or preferences about their treatment, and the role of shared decision-making in evidence-based practice.

By necessity our discussion of strategies for applying evidence to decision-making for individual patients, derived from decision-making research and teaching, is brief. Interested readers are directed to the further reading at the end of the chapter.

Does the evidence fit?

One of the first challenges in using evidence to help with decisions in practice is establishing that the research evidence is appropriate for the situation you are faced with.

In a series of studies examining nurses' decision-making in both primary care and acute care, Thompson et al (2001, 2004) produced a typology of the different types of decisions taken by nurses in practice that includes, amongst others, prevention, assessment, diagnostic, referral, intervention, timing, communication and service delivery type decisions (Table 8.1).

What this typology illustrates is that you are likely to be faced with a diversity of decisions in your everyday clinical practice and, consequently, a number of different types of questions for which you will need answers. There is a direct link between the decision problem you are faced with, the type of clinical question you are asking, and the type of research study design needed to help you answer the question and subsequently make your decision. A clinical scenario illustrates this linkage (Box 8.1). The point here is that if you can identify what type of decision you are making, it may help you to focus both your question and your search of the relevant literature.

As discussed in previous chapters, once you have identified relevant research evidence, you will need to reassure yourself of its validity and determine its usefulness for your individual patient. The latter involves assessing the similarity of (i) the context of the research study and your particular clinical environment, (ii) the patient group investigated in the study and the particular clinical circumstances of your patient and (iii) the application of the intervention/ investigation under study conditions and the intervention/ investigation that you plan to provide in your setting. At the end of this process, if you have determined that the research evidence is relevant to your particular decision

TABLE 8.1 DECISION TYPES, ASSOCIATED QUESTIONS AND EXAMPLES OF WHAT THEY LOOK LIKE IN PRACTICE. (FROM THOMPSON C, DOWDING D 2009 ESSENTIAL DECISION MAKING AND CLINICAL JUDGEMENT FOR NURSES. ELSEVIER, EDINBURGH, P.15)

Decision type	Clinical question	Example of what it looks like in practice
Intervention Decision that involves choosing among interventions	Treatment	Choosing a mattress for a frail elderly man who has been admitted with an acute bowel obstruction
Targeting A subcategory of intervention decisions, in the form of choosing which patient will benefit most from the intervention	Treatment	Deciding which patients should receive antiembolic stockings
Prevention Deciding which intervention is most likely to prevent occurrence of a particular health state or outcome	Treatment	Choosing which management strategy is likely to prevent recurrence of a healed leg ulcer
Timing Choosing the best time to deploy an intervention	Treatment	Choosing a time to begin asthma education for a newly diagnosed patient with asthma
Referral Decision to whom a patient's diagnosis or management should be referred	Treatment	Choosing that a patient's leg ulcer is arterial rather than venous and so merits medical rather than nursing management in the community

Communication Choosing how to communicate information to patients and relatives for maximum understanding. Also, choosing what information to communicate	Treatment (how to communicate) Prognostic (what to communicate, i.e. what is likely to happen in the future)	Choosing how to approach cardiac rehabilitation with an elderly patient who has had a myocardial infarction, whose family lives nearby and are worrying about her chances of having another heart attack
Service delivery, organisation and management Choosing how to configure service delivery or process	Treatment	Choosing how to organise handover so that communication is most effective
Assessment Decision that an assessment is required and/or what mode of assessment to use	Diagnostic and/or treatment	Choosing to use the Edinburgh Postnatal Screening Tool instead of an alternative instrument
Diagnosis Classifying signs and symptoms as a basis for a management or treatment strategy	Diagnostic	Deciding whether thrush or another cause is the reason for a woman's sore and cracked nipples
Information seeking The choice to seek (or not) further information before making a further clinical decision	Prognostic (what is likely to happen with no intervention or with intervention (i.e. wait versus decide)	Deciding that a guideline for monitoring patients who have had their ACE inhibitor dosage adjusted might be of use but choosing not to use it before asking a colleague
Experiential, understanding or 'hermeneutic' How to interpret cues in the process of care	Diagnostic uncertainty (but unlikely to be resolved using quantitative research)	Choosing how to reassure a patient who is worried about cardiac arrest after witnessing another patient arresting

---

BOX 8.1 The link between decisions, questions and study designs

Mr Smith is a 35-year-old man who has been referred to you for smoking cessation advice from the GP, after having had a nasty chest infection. The GP has advised him to try and stop smoking, and has suggested that he discusses his treatment options with you. A number of options are available to him, including the use of various types of nicotine replacement therapy and counselling programmes (both face to face and on the internet). He wants to know whether using an online resource would be as effective in helping him to stop smoking as some sort of face-to-face support (either individually or in a group) as he travels a lot and would find it difficult to keep a number of face-to-face appointments.

Type of decision: Intervention: involves choosing among alternatives
Type of clinical question: Effectiveness of a treatment
Type of study design: The optimum study design for a question about the effectiveness of a treatment is a systematic review of randomised controlled trials (RCTs) or a RCT.

---

scenario, you still have to try and incorporate it into your decision-making for this individual patient.

Strategies for decision-making

The majority of studies examining how nurses make decisions in practice suggest that they use a variety of different types of reasoning including hypothetico-deductive reasoning (e.g. Lamond et al 1996, Twycross & Powls 2006), heuristics and biases (Cioffi 1997), and intuition (e.g. King & Appleton 1997); depending on the clinical context and their own expertise. A brief description of each approach is given in Box 8.2. However, what characterizes these types of reasoning is the lack of any distinction between research evidence (i.e. the experiences of hundreds or even thousands of patients) and other kinds of evidence (such as a sense of intuitive 'correctness' in the course of action you are considering)

BOX 8.2 Types of clinical reasoning (based on theories of how people actually – rather than ought to – make decisions)

- Information processing: decision makers as active information seekers (or at least receivers of information), able to synthesise the information they are exposed to and make sense of it. A common mistake is to view reasoning as being 'like a computer'; [unlike a computer] decision makers have their processing 'bounded' (Simon & Zey 1992) by limited processing power, imperfect information, time constraints and other external factors.

- Hypothetico-deductive reasoning: decision-makers reason using stages. Perhaps the most well known being Elstein et al's (1978) proposal that clinical reasoning consists of 4 key stages: (a) cue acquisition in which clinical information is gathered, (b) hypothesis generation in which the clinician formulates ideas about what might be happening, (c) cue interpretation in which the meaning of the cues *given* the working hypotheses is established and (d) hypothesis evaluation in which the ideas of what might be happening are tested and either rejected or more information gathered.

- Intuitive judgement and decision-making: a very attractive label for nurse theorists and scholars. Intuition is itself contested, but commonly refers to variations of 'knowing without knowing quite why you know'. As knowledge, intuition is largely invisible and impossible to share with others (how can you share something when you don't know what it is you are sharing?). As a way of knowing, intuition is likely to draw on cognitive shortcuts (see below) called heuristics and the systematic errors that can result. Intuition can be a powerful tool in the hands of experts (Benner 1984; Benner & Tanner 1987).

- Heuristics (and their biases): decision makers rely on 'shortcuts' to handle complex information in decisions and this can result in predictable errors. By way of explanation, a person who is overconfident in the correctness of their knowledge, for example in their correctness in estimating risk, may have a false confidence in their ability to make accurate judgements and, as a result, may act inappropriately; they may fail to act when urgent action is required to mitigate the risk or may be overzealous in their actions (Thompson & Yang, 2009). Heuristic-based reasoning is often portrayed as a

(Continued)

BOX 8.2 Types of clinical reasoning (based on theories of how people actually – rather than ought to – make decisions)—Cont'd

negative phenomena; a positively orientated alternative is offered by fast and frugal reasoning presented below (Gigerenzer & Todd 1999).

- Fast and frugal reasoning: this approach suggests that the shortcuts we use (such as relying on the cues that you most recognise the value of when you are faced with a time-constrained judgement) often lead to good-quality judgements.
- The cognitive continuum: in this approach the reasoning style you employ is neither wholly rational nor wholly intuitive. Rather, the problem you are faced with determines (in part) the style of reasoning you employ (so a decision with no time constraints might be made using decision analysis, but the same decision with no time available will lead to intuitive reasoning).

---

as a basis for formulating decisions. Ignoring research (where it exists and is suitable) can lead to systematic errors or biases in reasoning and poor decision-making in practice.

In the rest of this section we explore approaches to decision-making that enable you explicitly to include research evidence in the decision process. These techniques are not all designed for scenarios where you need to take a decision quickly. However, if you have taken the time to ask a question, search for evidence and appraise it, it is worth expending the additional time to consider how to use the evidence effectively for your individual patient.

Using evidence in diagnostic decision-making

The process of diagnosis involves using the information we have collected about a patient's medical history, test results, signs and symptoms to try and identify what the cause of their current complaint may be (Thompson & Dowding 2009). Research evidence can provide information about the likelihood that an individual has a particular disease, as well as providing data on how accurate a diagnostic test is within a particular patient population. This section focuses on an approach, known as

Bayes' rule. Bayes is a set of rules for making sense of uncertain information in diagnostic decisions.

Bayes' rule or theorem can be described as:

The likelihood of patient X having a disease or condition (posterior probability)	=	the likelihood of patient X having disease or condition *before* you collected any evidence (prior probability)	x	the strenth of the evidence you have collected

Look at the example given in Box 8.3. To answer this woman's question, you would need to know:

- how likely it is that a 51-year-old woman has breast cancer (prior probability)
- the performance or accuracy of mammograms for identifying breast cancer in 51-year-old women (strength of evidence).

With this information you can then calculate what the likelihood is that the woman does actually have breast cancer (posterior probability). Before we look at the evidence, write down what you think the chances are that the woman has breast cancer, given your knowledge and experience.

Your learning from the previous chapters should stand you in good stead to identify the evidence needed to answer this question. We assume that you have used the PICO (population, intervention, comparison, outcome) approach to focus your question, have searched for the appropriate evidence, and are now faced with trying to specifically answer the woman's question. We have summarised the evidence we identified for the purposes of this example in Box 8.3.

We now have the components needed in Bayes' rule to calculate the likelihood or chance that, given a positive test result, your patient does actually have cancer. One of the easiest ways to do this is to use an online calculator such as the one found online at: http://araw.mede.uic.edu/cgi-bin/testcalc.pl (accessed May 11th 2010). You enter the prevalence of the disease condition (prior probability), which in this case is 262.4/100,000 or 0.003. You also

---

BOX 8.3 Using evidence in diagnosis

You are a primary care nurse practitioner. A 51-year-old woman who is attending clinic for her cervical smear test tells you that she had a mammogram two weeks ago. The test result has come back as 'suspicious' and she has been told that she now needs to go to the hospital for further tests. She asks you if this means she has cancer.

What is the likelihood that a 51-year-old woman has breast cancer?

According to cancer research UK (http://info.cancerresearchuk.org/prod_consump/groups/cr_common/@nre/@sta/documents/generalcontent/crukmig_1000ast-2843.xls), the incidence of breast cancer in women aged 50–54 is 262.4 per 100 000 population.

How good is a mammogram at detecting cancer in 51-year-old women?

Mammography has a sensitivity (chances of the test being positive, given that the patient has the condition) of between 75% and 95%, and a specificity (chances of the test being negative, given that the patient does not have the disease) of 94% to 97% (AHRQ screening for breast cancer, recommendation statement, 2009; accessed 11th May 2010, http://www.ahrq.gov/clinic/uspstf09/breastcancer/brcanrs.htm).

---

enter the sensitivity (0.75 to 0.95) and specificity (0.94 to 0.97). Given this information, the probability or likelihood of the woman having breast cancer (posterior probability) is calculated. Depending on how accurate the mammography screening (i.e. how good it is at detecting both positive and negative cases), the woman's probability of having breast cancer has risen to between 3% and 9%.

What this also indicates is the number of women who are 'false positives', in other words the number of women who have a positive test result despite not having the disease. The estimates for this particular test indicate between 1 in 11 and 1 in 29 women who have a positive mammogram actually have breast cancer. So, even though the woman described in Box 8.3 has had a positive test, and her chances of having breast cancer have increased, it is still more likely that it is a false alarm.

Using Bayes' rule can help us to evaluate how useful the signs and symptoms of particular diseases are for deciding if a patient has a given condition/disease; it helps determine the utility of diagnostic test results in particular groups of patients. It can also help you to determine if it is worthwhile carrying out a particular test for an individual patient. If the new information will not provide a greater insight into whether or not the patient either has or does not have the disease, it may not be worthwhile conducting the test. In instances such as the one described in Box 8.3, where there is a high chance of a false-positive test result, it may be worth discussing both the benefits and limitations of the test with the patient. The worry and additional testing associated with testing positive, for some patients, may outweigh the potential benefits provided by the test.

Using evidence in treatment decision-making

When we are discussing treatment decision-making, we are normally trying to decide which of a number of options (including doing nothing or 'watchful waiting') is the best approach for the patient; hopefully in collaboration with the patient. Research evidence can provide us with information about the comparative effectiveness of the different alternatives available, as well as their possible adverse or side effects. Often in health care there is no one 'obvious' alternative that is better than the others, perhaps due to the tradeoffs in terms of risks and benefits. The preferences and views of the individual patient are thus particularly important for helping inform what the best course of action may be. In these circumstances a more formal approach to decision-making, such as decision analysis, can help.

We will not guide you through the entire process of carrying out a decision analysis in this text (both Hunink et al (2001) and Dowding & Thompson (2009) provide a more detailed guide), but we do need to visit the principles of the approach. Decision analysis uses decision trees to structure the decision problem being faced, incorporates information from research evidence (in the form of probabilities or likelihood of certain events occurring) to the branches of the trees, and combines these with a formal evaluation of the patient's values or preferences (known as utility) for different outcomes, to reach an optimum decision.

To illustrate these principles, we use the example of a woman suffering from menopausal symptoms who needs to make a treatment decision.

In this example, the main clinical problem experienced by the woman is the hot flushes associated with menopause. The woman has been advised that lifestyle changes (increased physical activity and a healthy diet) as well as Hormone Replacement Therapy (HRT) may help to alleviate these symptoms. The possible outcomes of these interventions include: improvement or no improvement of hot flushes, development of breast cancer (HRT use may be associated with an increased risk of breast cancer) and protection against osteoporosis.

A decision tree helps to graphically display this information. As shown in Figure 8.1, the tree is easy to draw and should include: the problem (always shown to the left of the tree); the decision choices (represented by a square node), i.e. lifestyle changes alone

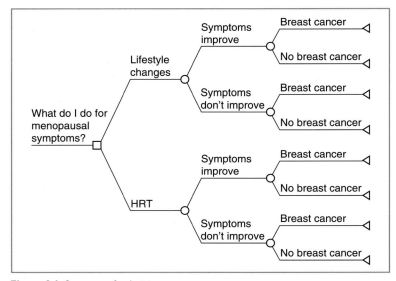

Figure 8.1 Structure of a decision tree

(comprising increased physical activity and a healthy diet) or the addition of HRT; and the possible 'chance' outcomes for each decision (represented by circle nodes), i.e. hot flushes improve or do not improve. For each of these chance branches, there are two further possible chance outcomes: development of breast cancer or no breast cancer. The chance outcome of osteoporosis or no osteoporosis is not shown on the tree, but it could easily be added.

Next, the probability of each of these outcomes occurring needs to be added to each branch of the tree as shown in Figure 8.2. Where it is available, high-quality research evidence, adapted for the individual patient's prognostic factors, can be used to give the probability or likelihood of certain events occurring. In the absence of research data, other estimations of likelihood (such as expert estimation) can be used, on the understanding that this type of evidence is less reliable than that derived from research. One of the key characteristics of research-derived probabilities is that they vary in samples and the populations to which they are applied, so measures of variability, extracted from the published research, are often helpful in decision analysis. For example, confidence intervals for the probabilities can be used to construct

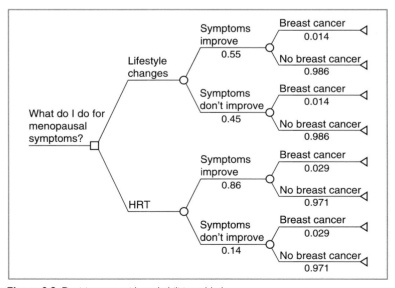

Figure 8.2 Decision tree with probabilities added

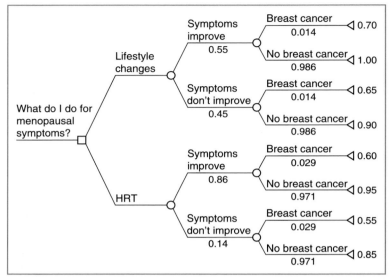

Figure 8.3 Decision tree with utilities added

upper and lower estimates for an individual and (later on in the process) the decision tested to see what happens to the optimal choice for an individual when the probabilities differ.

The final part of the decision tree entails evaluating patient's values, or utility, for the different outcomes (see following section) and adding this information to the tree. Utilities are usually expressed as a number between 0 (worst possible health state) and 1 or 100 (best possible health state), as shown in Figure 8.3. They are used as a measure of patient preference in the decision tree, and as such are a formal inclusion of patients' values into the decision process.

Once both probabilities and utilities are added into the tree, the best possible decision option is calculated. Probabilities and utilities for each decision branch are multiplied and then added together, until each decision option being considered has an overall number made up of the sum of all of its branches (Fig. 8.4). Here's how it is done:

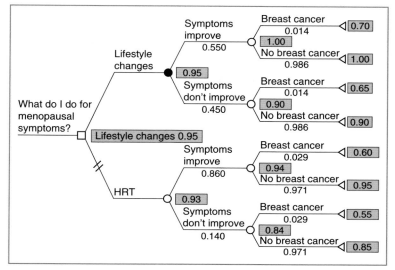

Figure 8.4 Decision tree with full calculations

Multiply the utility value for breast cancer at top right of tree (0.7) with the probability of that outcome (0.014) to yield 0.01.

For the branch below, multiply the utility value for no breast cancer (1.0) with the probability of that outcome (0.99, rounded up) to yield 0.99.

Add the resultant figures together to yield the expected utility for *hot flushes improved*: 0.01+ 0.99 = 1.0

Using the same formulae, carry out the calculations for the two branches of the chance node below to yield an expected utility for *hot flushes not improved*: 0.007+0.89= 0.9 (rounded up)

Working back to the left of the tree, calculate the overall expected utility for lifestyle changes: (1.0 × 0.55) + (0.9 × 0.45) = 0.95

Repeat this process to calculate the overall expected utility for HRT: = 0.93

Decision analysis assumes that individuals are rational, logical, decision-makers who will choose the decision option most likely to result in an outcome that has the greatest utility for the individual (Elwyn et al 2001). The decision option with the highest number is the one that maximises an individual's expected utility: i.e. is the option that is most likely to lead to an outcome that the individual decision maker values or prefers. In the decision tree in Figure 8.4, the best option for this particular woman is to change her lifestyle (expected utility of 0.95).

If the same decision scenario were given to a woman who wasn't as severely affected by hot flushes associated with the menopause and who, therefore, may have different values or utilities, this preferred option may change. The optimal decision may also change if the probability of different outcomes occurring was altered.

Decision analysis is not suitable for all healthcare decisions; it takes time and practice. But it can be a powerful tool for structuring decision problems, for formally ensuring that research evidence is incorporated into decisions about individual patients and that patients' values are explicitly considered and taken account of.

Evaluating patient preferences

A key component of an evidence-based decision is ascertaining how a patient feels about the potential risks and benefits associated with different treatment options available to them. Approaches for exploring patients' preferences vary in formality and aims. 'Value clarification exercises' are one way of helping patients clarify their own values to help them with a decision (O'Connor et al 2009). So, for example, a weigh scale, as shown in Figure 8.5, may be used to help the individual identify and assign weight to the pros and cons of different treatment options; in this example to aid an informed choice about HRT. Benefits and risks associated with the intervention are presented as 'weights' on the scale, with benefits, or reasons to choose the intervention, shown on the left, and risks, or reasons to forego

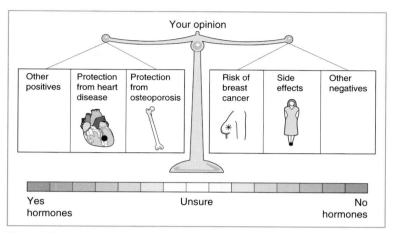

Figure 8.5 An example of a values clarification exercise designed to help women participate in decisions regarding hormone replacement therapy. Reproduced with permission from O'Connor et al 1999.

the intervention, shown on the right. The individual is asked to add any other reasons they can think of that may affect whether or not they would take HRT. They are then asked to indicate how important each risk and benefit is to them by shading or assigning stars to each 'weight' (completely shaded/5 stars = 'very important to me'; through to no shading/no stars = 'not at all important to me'). Having done this, they rate their predisposition towards taking HRT on the scale underneath, which is anchored between taking and not taking HRT, with being unsure in the middle (O'Connor et al 1999). The exercises can be used by patients to guide their decision processes, and by healthcare professionals as a reference point for ensuring that they understand what is important to the patient.

A patient's valuation of an outcome or health state (i.e. the utility they assign to a particular outcome) is usually expressed on a scale ranging from 'worst possible state of health' to 'best possible state of health'. As utility is an individual measure, it is possible that the worst and best possible health states will vary between individuals, as will their individual ratings of health states in between these two extremes. The simplest approach to formally assessing utility is to use a simple rating scale, where individuals are asked to rate outcomes on a scale from 0 (worst possible outcome) to 1 or 100 (best possible outcome). Other, more complex approaches include time trade off techniques, and a standard gamble (for further explanation of these approaches see Dowding & Thompson 2009).

Using utilities to measure patient preferences is not beyond criticism. The numbers associated with the utility for an outcome have been found to vary depending on the method used to generate them. Often, utility measures are carried out on a sample of individuals, and then assigned to an outcome within a decision analysis. These sample measures of utility may not be appropriate for individual patients, who may have different values and preferences to that represented by a group average. However, there is an argument to suggest that it is probably better to try and establish what a patient's values and preferences are for particular outcomes, either formally or informally, than not evaluate them at all (Elwyn et al 2001).

Shared decision-making

Gathering utilities and probabilities only really makes sense if – as a clinician – you are committed to working with the patients on the decisions that you both face. Aside from a general policy impetus (see for example the US preventative Services Task Force's assertion that patient–clinician partnership is 'central' to decision-making) (Sheridan et al 2004), there are also practical reasons why shared decision-making helps. First, patients who are involved in their decisions have better outcomes as a result (Coulter & Ellins 2007). Second, the factors that we think are important in decision-making (QALYs, functional ability, pain) may not be the same factors that drive a patient's choice. For an example of how wrong we can be (researchers and clinicians) the OMERACT initiative in arthritis (http://www.ncbi.nlm.nih.gov/pmc/articles/PMC2169260/?tool=pubmed) arose directly from a recognition that the outcomes we measure in clinical trials of treatments of rheumatoid arthritis (pain, mobility) are not the same outcomes that matter to patients with rheumatoid arthritis (fatigue is the one most commonly cited). The third, and perhaps most compelling reason for an evidence-based clinician, is that patients all vary in their preferences (and, indeed, the probability of events/outcomes associated with choices). This variability begs the question: how will you know what your patient's preferences are if you don't ask them? And if you ask them how will you know how to handle the information you get back?

As the majority of decisions that patients and professionals face together are intervention/treatment decisions (Thompson et al 2004) it is useful to consider at this juncture the different stages in the decision-making process and how patients might be involved. Entwistle and Watt (2009) put forward just such a model:

- In the information transfer stage of a decision in which the information necessary for informed consent for different treatment options is put forward, a shared approach recognises that this is a two way interaction: the professional provides the information perceived as required for patients to make a choice, whilst the patients express their preferences for the options they are presented with.

- At the deliberation stage of decision-making the clinician and the patient both consider what would be 'best' (in order to maximise utility, clinical outcome, a combination of both, or whatever criterion people use as a reference point for their decisions).

- Finally, at the choice/decision stage itself, both patient and professional actually commit to a decision option and its implementation.

This is a useful approach, but has its drawbacks; the main one being that it was developed from the treatment of women with breast cancer. In many circumstances (such as long-term conditions, co-morbid chronic illness, conditions on the margins of health and social care) the neatly defined treatment options, preferences and probabilities associated with some aspects of breast cancer care may not be present. In these circumstances nurses need to reflect on some broader considerations.

Before engaging in treatment discussions with the patient, the nurse can spend time 'structuring' or clarifying the decision problem. Questions to ask might include: what are the symptoms, concerns and potential diagnoses that need to be brought into play in any shared decision-making? Depending on the information I get back from the patient, what are the potential solutions I can offer (if any?). The aim here is not to curtail communication by framing the decision too tightly, rather to offer a start point for shared understanding between patient and professional.

After a choice has been made, then what? The reality is that for many patients there is not a single 'decision' followed by the 'treatment' working (or not). Furthermore, the nurse may have only minimal involvement in the patient's future management. Patients with chronic and long-term conditions often have to maintain active communication with nurses/doctors over some time. Decision-making is thus better viewed as a cyclical and iterative process rather than a single discrete event.

Thus far we have promoted shared decision-making as a positive force in the professional–patient partnership. Patients may benefit from feelings of greater control and autonomy – which constitute the necessary conditions for a happy life for all of us (Maslow 1954). Research studies suggest that patients value far more than clinical outcome alone when weighing up how much utility they get from a service or planned intervention (http://www.medicine.ox.ac.uk/bandolier/booth/glossary/QALY.html). They may also experience phenomena such as decisional conflict (whilst trying to weigh up possibly confusing and complex information) or regret once a decision has been made. Even 'good' decisions (Dowding & Thompson 2003) do not always work out and people often reflect on questions of 'what if'. Involving patients in a meaningful way in decision-making is also challenging for nurses. Revealing uncertainty and the limits of one's professional judgement and forecasting ability can feel uncomfortable. However, advice on the skills required for shared decision-making, and the associated competencies required for enacting them, does exist. Towle and Godolphin (1999) suggest that such skill sets should include:

- developing a partnership with patients
- establishing and reviewing patient preferences for information – including how much/little and the format most likely to lead to understanding
- establishing and reviewing preferences for the role that a patient would like to play in decision-making. Just as professionals vary in their attitudes to risk and desire for involvement and/or leadership, so do patients. Similarly, preferences for the degree of uncertainty associated with decisions that can be tolerated differ from person to person
- identifying and appropriately responding to concerns and expectations
- identifying choices (including those from patients) and the research evidence (weighted for its quality) associated with those choices
- directing patients to (or talking through) research, taking into account their preferences regarding information format and decision role
- negotiating decisions in partnership with the patient and helping resolving the conflicts that may arise
- developing and agreeing action plans and arrangements for follow-up/monitoring.

The above framework, which provides general guidance on sharing information and developing a shared understanding of the decision problem, can help you to involve patients in the decision process, as well as hopefully engage them with research evidence. To achieve this, you will also need to be able to fully explain the results of research studies to patients.

Explaining evidence to patients

If patients are to make informed decisions about their care, they will need to understand what the risks and benefits are of the different options available to them. Your role will be to take the evidence from different types of research studies and communicate it to patients either to help them evaluate their preferences for different options, or as a way of encouraging a more shared decision.

How we communicate information to patients can affect the decisions they take. Often when we are faced with healthcare decisions, we can look at potential outcomes in terms of likelihood of positive outcomes (such as survival) or negative outcomes (such as mortality). How we discuss these outcomes (known as 'framing') can have a significant impact on an individual's choice. Moxey et al (2003) carried out a systematic review of studies examining how framing affected decision choices. They found that when potential outcomes were expressed positively (e.g. survival) people were more likely to choose more invasive treatments such as surgery. In studies that looked at changes in health behaviour (such as weight loss, or stopping smoking) when potential outcomes were expressed in terms of gains to health, individuals were more likely to change their behaviour in the desired direction. Health professionals need to communicate the likelihood of different outcomes occurring to patients without unduly influencing their choices. To maintain an objective approach when communicating different options, information should be framed both positively and less positively.

How individuals understand risks and benefits differs, meaning that you may need to communicate the same information in different ways. Verbal descriptions, numerical presentations, and graphs and charts may all have a place in the communication of information to patients.

In general, it is probably better not to use verbal terms such as 'rarely' or 'sometimes' to explain the likelihood of outcomes occurring. This is because different individuals attach different meanings to the same verbal terms. A study by Timmermans et al (2004) found that doctors interpreted the verbal expression 'extremely rare' to mean that an event occurred in a range between 0% of the time and 15% of the time. Shaw and Dear (1990) showed that this spread of interpretations was not just a characteristic of professional interpretation but also extended to a mismatch in understanding between professionals and patients.

For this reason, it is generally better to try and communicate the potential risks and benefits associated with different treatment options using numerical or graphical means.

Numerical presentation of results of research studies include absolute risk, relative risk and number needed to treat. Absolute and relative risk can be communicated as percentages, probabilities or natural frequencies. Based on a number of studies examining the effect of different presentations of risk on an individual's understanding of risk (Covey 2007, Trevena et al 2006) it has been suggested that when communicating risk you should:

- use natural frequencies (e.g. this outcome occurs in 2 in a 100 people just like you) rather than probabilities (e.g. this outcome occurs in 0.02 people just like you)

- use absolute risk values (i.e. the observed or calculated risk or rate of an event occurring in a defined population) rather than relative risk values (which compare the risk or rate of an event in two different groups of people). For example, say: the risk of a non-smoking woman developing breast cancer is 1 in 100, rather than: there is a 50% increase in the risk of developing breast cancer if you smoke

- give an idea of the baseline level of risk where appropriate (e.g. the risk of you developing breast cancer over the next 10 years if you do not stop smoking is 2 in 100)

- use the same denominator across all the frequency information that you provide, so for example, if presenting data for two groups, use the denominator of 100 in both groups

(Dowding and Thompson 2009).

Many individuals have problems understanding numeric information so you may also need to consider providing information about risks and benefits graphically. The choice of graph you could use, and its applicability, depends on the type of information you are trying to convey (see Fig. 8.6 for examples). Stick figures or faces (icon displays) are useful for giving individuals information about their risk of developing a condition over time and how that risk may alter if they change their behaviour (Lipkus & Holland 1999). A good example of this approach is used by the risk calculator QRISK (www.qrisk.org), which uses information about your current health status to provide you with a risk of developing heart disease or stroke over 10 years.

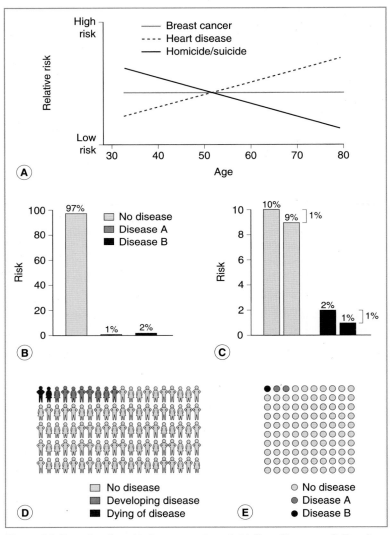

Figure 8.6 Examples of graphical representations of risk (from Thompson C, Dowding D 2009 Essential decision making and clinical judgement for nurses. Elsevier, Edinburgh, pp. 242–243).

This information is presented as a natural frequency, percentage and using an icon display. Other types of graphical display include bar graphs (for comparison of risk between groups), line graphs (for displaying information on risks of an event over time), pie charts (to show the proportion of individuals at risk of developing a condition) and risk ladders (for identifying the risk associated with different types of behaviour, anchored against reference points) (Lipkus & Holland 1999). How information is presented to individuals needs to be tailored both to their preferences and their ability to understand the information you are giving them. Note too, that the format that individuals may prefer may not necessarily be the format that enables them to fully understand the information they are being provided with (Ancker et al 2006).

Decision aids and decision support

One of the main ways in which research evidence can be used effectively to assist with decision-making, both for clinicians and for patients as a way of supporting through the process, is through the use of tools such as decision aids and decision support. It is important to distinguish between the two, as their focus and purpose differ. Decision support tools are normally developed for use by clinicians, whereas decision aids (see Box 8.4) are normally designed to be used by patients (either with or without clinician input). Both decision support tools

---

BOX 8.4 Main components of a Patient Decision Aid (O'Connor et al 2009)

- Provision of evidence-based information about health condition, the options, associated benefits, harms, probabilities and scientific uncertainties
- Assistance to help patients to recognise the values-sensitive nature of the decision and to clarify, either implicitly or explicitly, the value they place on the benefits, harms, and scientific uncertainties. Strategies that may be included in the decision aid are: describing the options in enough detail that clients can imagine what it is like to experience the physical, emotional, and social effects; and guiding clients to consider which benefits and harms are most important to them
- Provision of structured guidance in the steps of decision-making and communication of their informed values with others involved in the decision (e.g. clinician, family, friends)

and decision aids can be an effective way of helping to incorporate evidence from research into the decision process.

Clinical decision support tools can be paper or computer based. They incorporate evidence from research to provide clinicians with guidance for specific clinical decision. A systematic review of computerised decision support tools was carried out by Garg et al in 2005, which identified 100 studies that had evaluated the effectiveness of such tools in practice. The types of decisions they support include diagnosis, public health interventions (such as vaccination) and medication decisions. Decision support has perhaps had its greatest impact in the area of medications guidance, in particular, in preventing drug interactions and overdosing. The use of decision support tools in nursing is not common but is increasing. For instance, in England nurses who work for the telephone triage service NHS Direct use a decision support tool (based on protocols) to assist them with decision-making to provide advice to patients. The basic premise of many decision support tools is that evidence from research is incorporated into protocols which are then used to guide clinicians in appropriate practice. This is done via the use of guidance or alerts, which flag the clinician when they are deviating from recommended actions.

The evidence base for decision support in nursing is not as robust as that in medicine. A systematic review of the use of computerised decision support in nursing (Randell et al 2007) found very few studies that had formally evaluated the effect of such tools on outcomes for patients. These studies suggested that the effect of such tools was equivocal, with some positive benefits, but also some potential negative impacts on practice and outcomes. If decision support tools are developed to help nurses with evidence-based practice, their impact should be evaluated effectively.

In contrast, decision aids are resources specifically designed to help patients to make choices regarding the treatment options where there is no one obvious 'best' option (O'Connor et al 2009). They can be used within consultations with clinicians, or as an additional resource to help with the decision process (Entwistle & Watt 2009). A systematic review of the impact of decision aids on patient decision-making suggests that the aids can improve knowledge, reduce the amount of conflict patients feel about the decision process and help individuals to reach a decision (O'Connor et al 2009). When decision aids incorporate specific information about the probabilities related to outcomes, they improve the accuracy of individuals' risk perceptions (O'Connor et al 2009). The use of decision aids may also impact on the types of choices that patients make, such as reducing invasive surgery, and reducing PSA screening (O'Connor et al 2009).

Decision aids vary in the information they contain and their quality. In an attempt to try and help patients and healthcare professionals evaluate decision aids; the International Patient Decision Aid Standards (IPDAS) Collaboration has produced a list of standards (http://ipdas.ohri.ca/). If you are interested in trying to locate a decision aid for a particular condition, there is an online inventory of patient decision aids at http://decision-aid.ohri.ca/AZinvent.php.

Summary

In this chapter we have given a flavour of various ways in which research evidence from studies on populations can be integrated into decision-making for individual patients. It is important to highlight that the evidence from research is often only one of many factors that need to be taken into account when making healthcare decisions, and that issues such as patient preferences, and ensuring that patients are included in the decision process, are equally important issues to address wherever appropriate. We encourage the interested reader to undertake more in-depth reading using the resources listed, and to practice using decision support tools. We also encourage the reader to consolidate their learning from this chapter by undertaking the online exercises (see website)

References

Ancker, J., Senathirajah, Y., Kukafka, R., et al., 2006. Design features of graphs in health risk communication: A systematic review. J. Am. Med. Inform. Assoc. 13, 608–618.

Benner, P., 1984. From novice to expert: excellence and power in clinical nursing practice. Addison-Wesley, Reading, Mass.

Benner, P., Tanner, C., 1987. How expert nurses use intuition. Am. J. Nurs. 87 (1), 23–31.

Cioffi, J., 1997. Heuristics, servants to intuition in clinical decision making. J. Adv. Nurs. 26, 203–208.

Coulter, A., Ellins, J., 2007. Effectiveness of strategies for informing, educating, and involving patients. Br. Med. J. 335, 2427.

Covey, J., 2007. A meta-analysis of the effects of presenting treatment benefits in different formats. Med. Decis. Making 27, 638–654.

DiCenso, A., Cullum, N., Ciliska, D., 1998. Implementing evidence based nursing: some misconceptions. Evid. Based Nurs. 1, 38–39.

Dowding, D., Thompson, C., 2003. Measuring the quality of judgement and decision-making in nursing. J. Adv. Nurs. 44 (1), 49–57.

Dowding, D., Thompson, C., 2009. Evidence based decisions: the role of decision analysis. In: Thompson, C., Dowding, D. (Eds.), Essential decision making and judgement for nurses. Elsevier, Edinburgh, pp. 173–196.

Elstein, A.S., Shulman, L.S., Sprafka, S.A., 1978. Medical problem solving: an analysis of clinical reasoning. Harvard University Press, Cambridge, MA.

Elwyn, G., Edwards, A., Eccles, M., et al., 2001. Decision analysis in patient care. Lancet 358, 571 Cambridge, MA: 574.

Entwistle, V., Watt, I., 2009. Involving patients in decision making. In: Thompson, C., Dowding, D. (Eds.), Essential decision making and judgement for nurses. Elsevier, Edinburgh, pp. 217–234.

Field, P.A., 1987. The impact of nursing theory on the clinical decision-making process. J. Adv. Nurs. 12, 563–571.

Garg, A., Ahikari, N., McDonald, H., et al., 2005. Effects of computerized clinical decision support systems on practitioner performance and patient outcomes: a systematic review. JAMA 293 (10), 1223–1238.

Gigerenzer, G., Todd, P., 1999. Simple heuristics that make us smart. Oxford University Press, New York.

Grobe, S.J., Drew, J.A., Fonteyn, M.E., 1991. A descriptive analysis of experienced nurses' clinical reasoning during a planning task. Res. Nurs. Health 14, 305–314.

Hunink, M., Glasziou, P., Siegel, J., et al., 2001. Decision making in health and medicine. Integrating evidence and values. Cambridge University Press, Cambridge.

Itano, J.K., 1989. A comparison of the clinical judgment process in experienced registered nurses and student nurses. J. Nurs. Educ. 28 (3), 120–126.

King, L., Appleton, J.V., 1997. Intuition: a critical review of the research and rhetoric. J. Adv. Nurs. 26, 194–202.

Lamond, D., Crow, R., Chase, J., 1996. Judgements and processes in care decisions in acute medical and surgical wards. J. Eval. Clin. Pract. 2 (3), 211–216.

Lipkus, I., Hollands, J., 1999. The visual communication of risk. J. Natl. Cancer Inst. Monogr. 25, 149–163.

Maslow, A., 1954. Motivation and personality. Harper and Row New York, New York.

Moxey, A., O'Connell, D., McGettigan, P., 2003. Describing treatment effects to patients. How they are expressed makes a difference. J. Gen. Intern. Med. 18, 959.

O'Connor, A.M., Bennett, C.L., Stacey, D., et al., 2009. Decision aids for people facing health treatment or screening decisions. Cochrane Database Syst. Rev. (3). Art. No.: CD001431. doi:10.1002/14651858.CD001431.pub2.

O'Connor, A., Wells, G., Tugwell, P., et al., 1999. The effects of an 'explicit' values clarification exercise in a woman's decision aid regarding postmenopausal hormone therapy. Health Expect. 2 (1), 21–32.

Randell, R., Mitchell, N., Dowding, D., Cullum, N., Thompson, C., 2007. Effects of computerised decision support systems on nursing performance and patient outcomes: a systematic review. J. Health Serv. Res. Policy 12 (4), 242–251.

Shaw, N.J., Dear, P.R., 1990. How do parents of babies interpret qualitative expressions of probability? Arch. Dis. Child. 65 (5), 520–523.

Sheridan, S.L., Harris, R.P., Woolf, S.H., 2004. Shared decision making about screening and chemoprevention. Am. J. Prev. Med. 26, 56–66.

Simon, H., Zey, M., 1992. Decision making and problem solving. Decision making: alternatives to rational choice models. Sage, Newbury Park: CA, pp. 32–53.

Thompson, C., Dowding, D., 2009. Essential decision making and judgement for nurses. Elsevier, Edinburgh.

Thompson, C., Yang, H., 2009. Nurses' decisions, irreducible uncertainty and maximising nurses' contribution to patient safety. Healthc. Q. 12 (SP), e178–e185.

Thompson, C., McCaughan, D., Cullum, N., et al., 2001. Research information in nurses' clinical decision making: what is useful? J. Adv. Nurs. 36, 376–388.

Thompson, C., Cullum N McCaughan, D., Sheldon, T., Raynor, P., 2004. Nurses, information use, and clinical decision making--the real world potential for evidence-based decisions in nursing. Evid. Based Nurs. 7 (3), 68–72.

Timmermans, D., Molewijk, B., Stigglebout, A., et al., 2004. Different formats for communicating surgical risks to patients and the effect on choice of treatment. Patient Educ. Couns. 54, 255–263.

Towle, A., Godolphin, W., 1999. Framework for Teaching and learning informed shared decision making? Br. Med. J. 319, 766–771.

Trevena, L., Davey, H., Baratt, A., et al., 2006. A systematic review on communicating with patients about evidence. J. Eval. Clin. Pract. 12, 13–23.

Twycross, A., Powls, L., 2006. How do children's nurses make clinical decisions? Two preliminary studies. J. Clin. Nurs. 15, 1324–1335.

Further Reading/Internet Resources

Gigerenzer, G., 2002. Reckoning with risk: learning to live with uncertainty. Penguin, London.

An easy to read introduction into the fallibility of human reasoning and how to interpret research evidence.

Hunink, M., Glasziou, P., Siegel, J., et al., 2001. Decision making in health and medicine. Integrating evidence and values. Cambridge University Press, Cambridge.

A good overview of the process of decision analysis.

Thompson, C., Dowding, D., 2009. Essential decision making and clinical judgement for nurses. Elsevier, Edinburgh.

More detailed discussion of the issues raised here, as well as an overview of decision making in nursing.

Online Inventory of Patient Decision Aids can be found at: http://decisionaid.ohri.ca/AZinvent.php.

Online calculator for Bayes' theorem: http://araw.mede.uic.edu/cgi-bin/testcalc.pl.

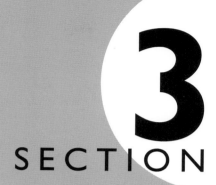

SECTION 3

The process of changing practice

CHAPTER 9

Using research evidence to change how services are delivered

Lin Perry

KEY POINTS

- Any change in practice requires commitment, effort and 'buy-in' from practitioners and managers. There may be training, cost and time implications.

- Meticulous planning and preparation is essential and frameworks are available to aid this.

- Consideration of the wider picture is important, for example gaining an understanding of the organisational culture, will pay dividends.

- Core elements of an evidence-based service change include:
  - **identifying** the practice(s) that need to change by, for example, having a baseline measure of current practice, identifying the 'evidence–practice gap', targeting the particular local change priority/need
  - **planning** for change: understanding the organisational environment and local culture, identifying the senior person to sponsor high-level support, recruiting local champions, engaging the grass-roots workforce, seeking users' views and involvement, identifying likely supports/supporters and recruiting them, identifying likely barriers/hurdles and developing strategies to address them, agreeing measures to demonstrate change, identifying the technical and humanistic approaches and activities required to prepare for and effect change, considering ways to ensure changes will be sustainable
  - **implementing** the service/practice change using the agreed methods
  - **studying** the change processes as they progress, communicating and fine-tuning these as required, comparing baseline and repeated measures
  - **evaluating** the processes and outcomes achieved, consolidating and maximising sustainability and deciding on next steps.

Introduction

The aim of this chapter is to help nurses understand how different types of evidence can be applied to effect changes in how services are provided. It sets out a range of approaches commonly used to structure service and practice change initiatives. Clinical projects that have focused on development of healthcare services in a variety of settings and locations are used as illustrations. These include:

- the <u>E</u>ncouraging <u>B</u>est <u>P</u>ractice in <u>R</u>esidential <u>A</u>ged <u>C</u>are Nutrition and Hydration project (EBPRAC), undertaken within care homes of two not-for-profit provider organisations across New South Wales, Australia

- the Young adult OUtReach project for people with type I Diabetes Mellitus in rural areas (YOUR-Diabetes), conducted in sites across New South Wales Australia
- the initial site studies of the Essentials of Care Emancipatory Practice Development (EoC e-PD) programme from an acute hospital in metropolitan Sydney
- a Total Knee Replacement pathway redesign programme (TKR2) from a major acute hospital
- two London based projects: STEP1, the multi-site South Thames Evidence-based Practice project and STEP2, the Stroke Treatment for Every Person project (STEP2) undertaken in an acute tertiary hospital.

These projects between them involved nurses, nursing assistants, medical staff, allied health professionals, patients and families and spanned a wide range of settings. Thus they involve many of the key stakeholders and locations by whom and in which health services are developed and delivered. The message here is that evidence-based changes to service provision or structure need not be restricted to any specific area of practice, clinical or professional group. Most topics have varied evidence bases, and each clinical setting presents its own challenges. Lessons of success and good practice are available from all contexts and environments.

How is this relevant to me?

Lessons learned from each of these projects have direct relevance for healthcare practitioners and for clinical governance/effectiveness leads charged with implementing service developments. The diversity of project topics, settings (including critical care, acute and rehabilitation wards, mental health services, outpatient and day centres, general practice, community, domiciliary and aged care locations), geographical locations across two continents, from metropolitan and urban to rural environments, and participants from diverse healthcare professional backgrounds has produced a wealth of information about what worked in which contexts.

For those embarking upon or contemplating changing service provision, this chapter offers an illustrated 'basic steps' approach. It starts with an overview of some commonly quoted approaches to change (such as Continuous Quality Improvement), teases out barriers to change, and then considers key steps for effecting service change. It flags pragmatic frameworks and checklists that can give structure to the change process, and supplies examples and explanations for what has/not worked, allowing readers to make comparisons with their own environments.

Approaches to changing services

Implementation of evidence-based changes in clinical practice is a fast-growing field of professional science. It has grown from early, somewhat mechanistic conceptualisation as guideline development and delivery and audit, to encompass learning from quality improvement programmes and a variety of psychological and organisational approaches, in recognition of the complexity of healthcare systems. A Cochrane group has been established to collate relevant systematic reviews (the Cochrane Effective Practice and Organisation of Care Group: http://epoc. cochrane.org/) and a new terminology created; Straus et al (2009) refer to 90 terms and permutations of language applying to the process which they define as 'the methods for closing the gaps from knowledge to practice': knowledge transfer or translation (KT), or knowledge-to-action (K2A).

As will be discussed in Chapter 10, the implementation of any change in service is affected by, impacts on, and is intertwined with organisational culture. A brief consideration of three approaches or models for change that take account of context issues follows.

Quality improvement (QI)

Early QI initiatives within health care followed their development within the business world. The Total Quality Movement from Toyota and the achievements of British Airways and Xerox are commonly cited examples. From the late 1980s local quality initiatives became increasingly common in nursing, described, for example, as Quality Circles or CQI (Continuous Quality Improvement). Two reports, from the US (Kohn et al 1999) and the UK (Department of Health 2000a) are often credited with being the catalysts to major programmes of healthcare quality improvement in these countries. In the US, the report 'To Err is Human: Building a Safer Health System' was followed in 2001 by 'Crossing the Quality Chasm: A New Health System for the 21st Century'; these inspired the Institute for Healthcare Improvement (IHI) '100 000 Lives' Campaign, which by 2006 was claimed to have prevented an estimated 124 000 deaths through patient-safety initiatives, and the subsequent 5 Million Lives Campaign. IHI currently has an internationally acclaimed suite of research implementation and healthcare QI initiatives and tools, some freely available, through its website http://www.ihi.org/ihi (see Table 9.1 on the website). In the UK, the 'Organisation with a Memory' report (Department of Health 2000a) was followed by a series of initiatives from the Department of Health: the NHS Modernisation Agency, for example, developed a range of written resources to support QI and ran topic-specific improvement courses. Superseded by the NHS Institute for Innovation and Improvement (http://www.institute.nhs.uk/innovation/innovation/introduction.html), this institute continues to provide resources and a programme of QI initiatives.

A wide range of QI frameworks has been developed. Lean Thinking, which emphasises pursuing perfection in terms of: right patient, right place, on time, every time, helping people recognise and intervene when things are going wrong (Westwood et al 2007; www.institute.nhs.uk/ServiceTransformation/Lean+Thinking), is just one example. Continuous improvement is through enhancing the patient journey and eliminating waste. Simple aids such as the TIMWOODS acronym and 5S Process can help with identification and elimination of waste (Boxes 9.1 and 9.2).

Further examples of QI approaches, described in terms of their key stages, can be viewed on the website (Table 9.2). Permutations of the Plan, Do, Study, Act (PDSA) cycles are incorporated in some of these approaches(http://www.institute.nhs.uk/quality_and_service:improvement_tools/quality_and_service:improvement_tools/plan_do_study_act.html; Fig. 9.1).

The TKR2 project utilised PDSA cycles to test and refine a series of changes to the patient pathway, including development of a pre-assessment clinic, new information leaflets, earlier and more intensive training in crutch-walking by physiotherapists. Participants appreciated the chance to trial changes incrementally, with first cycles involving small numbers of patients. Changes could be fine-tuned rapidly, so progress occurred with minimal delay (Lucas 2008).

BOX 9.1 TIMWOODS for Lean Thinking: domains in which waste may occur

- **T**ransportation, with excessive carriage of people and goods across locations
- **I**nventory, with unnecessary accumulation of stores and goods, the ideal being 'Just In Time' delivery and minimal stock levels
- **M**otion, representing wasted activity
- **W**aiting, being as much a waste of time for patients as staff
- **O**verproduction, resulting in unused resource
- **O**ver-processing, being as much an issue for care processes as products
- **D**efects and errors, the processes that produced them and the work required to rectify them
- **S**taff under-utilisation, resulting in loss of skills, demotivation and lost productivity

BOX 9.2 Five S: A lean process to eliminate waste

- **Sort** – essential items and clutter
- **Set in order** – organise work area around processes/processes around the work required
- **Shine** – set in order processes to maintain equipment, etc., in functional order
- **Standardisation** – of processes, etc., across the organisation
- **Sustain** – make part of everyday work, monitor

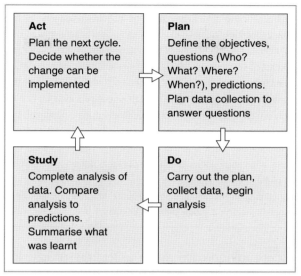

Figure 9.1 The four stages of the PDSA cycle: Plan - the change to be tested or implemented **Do** - carry out the test or change **Study** - data before and after the change and reflect on what was learned **Act** – plan the next change cycle or full implementation (adapted from http://www.institute.nhs.uk/quality_and_service_improvement_tools/quality_and_service_improvement_tools/plan_do_study_act.html)

Action research

Action research (AR) in healthcare has been defined as:

a period of inquiry that describes, interprets and explains social situations while executing a change intervention aimed at improvement and involvement. It is problem-focused, context-specific and future-orientated. Action research is a group activity with an explicit critical value basis and is founded on a partnership between action researchers and participants, all of whom are involved in the change process. The participatory process is educative and empowering, involving a dynamic approach in which problem identification, planning, action and evaluation are interlinked. Knowledge may be advanced through reflection and research, and qualitative and quantitative research methods may be employed. (Waterman et al 2001, 11).

BOX 9.3 Defining characteristics of action research
(Hart & Bond 1995, p.37–38)

Action research:
1. is educative
2. deals with individuals as members of social groups
3. is problem focused, context-specific and future orientated
4. involves a change intervention
5. aims at improvement and involvement
6. involves a cyclic process in which research, action and evaluation are interlinked
7. is founded on a research relationship in which those involved are participants in the change process

---

AR represents an approach to the generation of new knowledge rather than a specific research method (Meyer 2000). In short, it enables participants to generate solutions to practical problems whilst providing a means for their professional development: practitioners research their own practice or the practice of others, or an outside researcher is engaged to help them identify problems, seek and implement practical solutions and systematically monitor and reflect on the processes and outcomes of change. AR proceeds through cycles of action and reflection. A typology developed by Hart and Bond (1995) lists seven distinguishing criteria (Box 9.3).

The STEP2 project used AR. It developed as an organisational problem solving response, and as a professional aspiration to implement more explicitly research-based practice. Led by an insider-researcher who developed a strongly collaborative role with participants, it employed a variety of educative and evaluative approaches focused on understanding how to develop individuals and professional groups into a unitary cohesive stroke team.

Practice development in nursing

Practice development (PD) as a specific activity has been a recognised feature of nursing for several decades. In general, it encompasses a variety of philosophical approaches and processes with a common core of on-going commitment to achievement of demonstrable improvements in care processes and patient outcomes. In 1999, McCormack et al summarised the approach that had grown out of the work of the Royal College of Nursing Institute in a definition of PD as,

...a continuous process of improvement towards increased effectiveness in person-centred care, through the enabling of nurses and health care teams to transform the culture and context of care.

Nursing PD has developed alongside and from streams of work including quality initiatives, conceptual developments focused on nursing care models, the nursing process, nurse decision-making and nursing competency frameworks. PD approaches pay equal heed to the environment in which practice occurs at policy, strategic, operational and cultural levels. This entails attending to characters, characteristics and features of the local setting, to achieve as full an understanding as possible of the relationships and meaning that it encompasses for those who work in it and are cared for within it. McCormack et al (2007a and b) provide a framework to help understand this: **'What'** is the PD activity and **'Why'** is it being established; **'Who'** is it for – whose practice is being developed, what is their level of involvement, what is the scale of the activity, what is the context and what is the culture and the leadership in their environment; **'By whom'** is it being developed – how are they involved and what is their theoretical and working relationship with participants; and **'How'** does learning and change happen – how is knowledge generated and used?

Similarly, a framework such as the PARiHS framework (Promoting Action on Research Implementation in Health Services, Rycroft-Malone et al 2002) can aid adequate preparation for service change by prompting consideration of (i) the characteristics of the evidence underpinning the proposed change, be it research, experiential and/or other evidence; (ii) the context within which the change will happen; and (iii) the characteristics of change facilitators including their roles, skills, attributes and availability (Fig. 9.2). In terms of the context for change, PARiHS flags

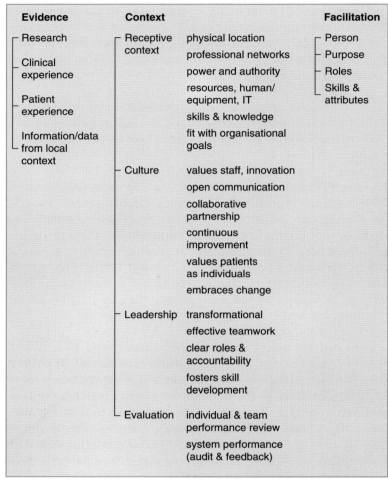

Figure 9.2 The PARIHS framework (Promoting Action on Research Implementation in Health Services) (adapted from Rycroft-Malone et al 2002)

the importance of local culture and leadership: staff values; their attitudes to innovation and continuous improvement; the degree to which they foster open communication and embrace change; and the degree to which leaders use transformational versus traditional control styles. These aspects all affect how practitioners experience accountability for their actions and how they develop as individuals and advance their skills. Ultimately this influences the effectiveness of teamwork. The availability and application of evaluation processes are also important, including the functionality of individual, team and system performance review. Altogether these features affect the receptiveness of the environment to change.

PARiHS was employed in the EBPRAC project to examine the contexts and cultures of the care homes as sites to implement evidence-based change. Features unique to this setting, such as their simultaneous function as resident homes, staff workplaces and small-medium sized businesses, and the particular role and function of Registered Nurses in this environment, were revealed. Understandings provided through application of this structured form of inquiry were invaluable to the change process (Perry et al 2010a).

Attitudes and barriers to using research evidence

Any change in service delivery requires commitment from practitioners and their managers so careful consideration as to how the proposal may be received and the prevailing attitude towards evidence informing the change is important. The next section emphasises the point that evidence 'chosen' by nurses to inform their nursing decision-making comprises a variety of elements and derives from a number of sources, not always the sources or routes preferred by project managers trying to effect an evidence-based change.

Nursing knowledge

The concepts, definitions and relationships between information, evidence and knowledge for nursing continue to be debated and further reading is available (for example, Benner 1984, Bonis 2009, Carper 1978, Mantzoukas & Jasper 2007, Porter & O'Halloran 2008). Nursing 'knowledge' is broadly based, derived from a wide variety of sources of information. The novice nurse works consciously and analytically, learning to recognise situations in which particular aspects of theoretical knowledge apply, thus developing practical knowledge that extends and refines their textbook knowledge, eventually enabling recognition of clinical states without conscious deliberation (Tanner 2006). For many nurses, explicit consideration of research evidence does not figure highly.

Attitudes to use of evidence have been extensively explored using the BARRIERS Scale to assess:

- nurses' research values, research skills and awareness
- nurses' perceptions of limitations imposed by the work environment
- the research itself, its qualities, presentation and accessibility.

Collating findings from 53 studies that employed this scale, Kajermo et al (2010), demonstrated that nurses perceived difficulties arising from all these areas. Across these studies, the barriers most consistently highly ranked featured the inaccessibility of evidence (whether due to incomprehensible statistics, poorly synthesised or publicised findings), nurses' research skill deficits, and lack of authority, resources and support to effect change.

Preliminary analyses from three of the nine care homes that took part in the EBPRAC project reported that only two participants, both managers, explicitly identified research as a foundation of care. Guidelines were acknowledged but, importantly, if, in the process of implementing guidelines, people were expected to abandon what they had previously believed to be the right thing to do, the underpinning research had to be credible to them. Some went even further and needed to see that what was presented was not just workable but actually worked before they would engage with it. The worth of any change rested on how it was experienced in practice, how it was applied and what it was seen to achieve, rather than any intrinsic or scientific merit (Perry et al 2010a).

More fundamentally, nursing knowledge is shaped by nurses' philosophical disposition, i.e. their values. Often unspoken and, possibly, unrecognised values profoundly influence what nurses attend to in any particular situation and the options they consider and act upon.

Knowing the patient, client or resident

In the EBPRAC project, both participant organisations espoused values of person-centred care. Staff interviews reflected the centrality of residents' experiences as an evidence source. Staff talked about seeking and knowing the preferences of the individual, about respect for the individuality and personhood of each resident and, in regional areas where staff and residents came from the same small local communities, staff considered residents as like family and were able to see themselves in their situation. On-the-job, daily interactions with residents enabled close knowledge of the residents as individuals, which meant that staff felt they just knew what to do: 'I see them every day, 5 days a week, so you think you tend to know' (Perry et al 2010a).

Central to nursing knowledge is their knowledge of the patient. Tanner (2006) cites a number of studies that describe nurses' understanding of their patients. This knowledge derives from working with patients, hearing their accounts of their illness experience, observing them (more than just 'doing the obs'), coming to know them as a person and understanding how they typically respond. Accessing this form of evidence may not entail conscious thought for most experienced nurses.

Clinical experience

Spenceley et al (2008) reported that nurses prefer to use people (peers and other nurses) as information sources. Thompson et al (2004) reported that accessibility and usefulness were viewed as primary attributes for sources of information; hence, experiential sources of information such as nurse specialists or experienced colleagues were the preferred information sources. The 'useful' nature of information from nurse specialists and colleagues derived from its grounding in clinical reality and experience. Little wonder, then, that clinicians at hand are often the preferred source of evidence. The downside is that the information received may represent the personal opinion of the author, unsupported by other evidence, which is the least reliable and valid form of evidence (Thompson 2003).

Key components of service change

A common feature of the approaches to change highlighted earlier is the importance of taking a systematic and measured approach to transferring healthcare evidence or knowledge into practice (knowledge transfer). The frameworks described earlier, such as those used in quality improvement or practice development, have a role here. A further example is the Knowledge Transfer Framework for Research Users devised by Ward et al (2010), which comprises detailed questions to be considered when integrating knowledge transfer into day-to-day tasks, with questions being grouped by:

- problem
- context
- knowledge
- intervention
- use.

The next section is structured using these headings so that interested readers can, at the same time as reading this section, take account of the comprehensive and probing questions of the Knowledge Transfer Framework for Research Users (available at http://www.leeds.ac.uk/lihs/psychiatry/research/ TransferringKnowledgeIntoAction/documents/Knowledge%20 Brokering%20Final%20report.pdf, Appendix D).

Identifying the problem

Identifying appropriate topics

If you always do what you've always done, you'll always get what you always got.

This statement neatly represents the first step in changing practice or a service – acknowledging the need to change the processes, procedures and practices in order to change the outcomes. It is seldom realistic to expect that a personal 'Eureka' moment will be shared by everyone involved, but one small step for one person can represent the start of a giant leap for an organisation.

The initial idea may come about as a local response to local practice issues, often in relation to perceptions or reports of quality of care. This was the case with the EBPRAC project, where 'nutrition teams' in care homes identified the nutritional priority issues for their site, using a variety of formally gathered information: audits of care plans, nutritional assessments of residents, interview data and discussion groups with residents and families and with staff, resident food satisfaction surveys, analysis of weighed food and records of residents' dietary intake to name a few. For one of the STEP1 projects, patients' dissatisfaction with current nutritional practices was made apparent in letters of complaint (ACHCEW 1997). For the YOuR-Diabetes project, the impetus came from clinicians' dissatisfaction with what they were able to achieve for their clients, brought into focus by a report which detailed metropolitan compared to rural service provision (Lister & Brodie 2008). Funding enabled a group of clinicians and researchers to initiate a formal consultation process which provided information about the experiences of young people with type 1 Diabetes Mellitus accessing adult services in rural locations, the difficulties and barriers they encountered, and what sort of services they thought could meet their needs (Perry et al 2008).

Service and practice development may also occur in response to high level strategic initiatives or directives. In a national audit, one major London teaching hospital found itself scored in the bottom quartile in the country for its treatment of stroke. Occurring alongside a local campaign for change, the response was a rapid and radical redesign project to create a dedicated stroke service – STEP2 (Kilbride et al 2010).

Who benefits?

It is sometimes not enough that the literature identifies benefits for patients; clinicians have to be persuaded that these benefits will accrue for their patients and be worth the time and trouble that changing working practices entails. In one of the STEP1 projects, O'Tuathail et al (2000, p.27) implemented standardised multidisciplinary assessment for older people prior to discharge. One individual was concerned that the screening tool might identify clinical depression where patients were experiencing distress accompanying ill health and removal from their home environment and result in unnecessary medication. Taking time to understand the problems indicated a way forward: having the individual train a trusted nurse to undertake depression screening resolved the impasse.

Local and national opinion

Any changes envisaged need to be congruent with the objectives of the organisation and accepted as a current priority. For STEP2, when national audit results were released, clinical staff dissatisfaction with services was matched by that of board members. The EoC e-PD project developed from concerns of a small group of nurses in one hospital about patient safety issues with nursing shortages and reduced skill and experience levels at the bedside (Clarke et al 2010). However, when similar concerns were reported during a major inquiry (Special Commission of Inquiry 2008), a wider programme using the principles of this local development was advocated. With this recommendation accepted by government, other hospitals implemented EoC e-PD as local responses to a strategic directive. Aligning concerns can build a coalition for change.

Understanding the context for change

A situation/diagnostic analysis is crucial to discovering those organisational, personal and interpersonal characteristics that will be relevant to transferring knowledge into action in this setting. This needs to be achieved before or alongside early project planning stages. The PARiHS framework (Fig. 9.2) or that from Ward et al (2010) can be employed for this purpose.

The organisational environment

Organisational elements that can positively influence the progress of a project include the presence of strong leadership and good managerial relations reflected in attitudes that support trying new approaches and taking risks. These elements should be allied with professional support networks and effective audit and feedback systems to keep people abreast of progress (Greenhalgh et al 2004). Organisational stability is also important; of the nine trusts involved in the STEP1 project, three underwent major reorganisation or merger within the life of the project, two within the first 6 months. A period of organisational change may not be the best time to seek support for changes in practice; at the very least, practice changes must be planned to take other changes into account (Bignell et al 2000, pp. 9–10). Reports of 'change overload' and low appetite or tolerance for more change are common (Doherty et al 2000, p.14; Perry et al 2010a), however, it is worth bearing in mind that perceptions of change may vary according to management and presentation.

It is essential to consider how the change relates to the organisation's priorities, structures and strategic plans, and the change agent must have a good grasp of these. Ways of achieving this include reviewing public reports, human resources information, clinical audits, minutes of key group meetings (e.g. of trust board, departmental heads, charge nurses), observation of meetings, interviews, focus groups and informal discussions with key figures. If the selected topic fits within an identified priority area, high-level support may be easier to recruit. The better the 'fit' between the change initiative and existing priorities and structures, the less time and effort required to introduce it and perhaps the greater the likelihood of success (Miller et al 1999).

Local culture: 'the way we do things round here'

This entails putting together a picture of organisational culture at team, ward or unit level as well as trust-wide. Most nurses will be familiar with the marked differences in character encountered even between adjacent wards sharing consultants and patient intake. As 'incomers', Perry et al (2000, p.17) used the Assessment of Ward Environment Schedule (Nolan et al 1998) to gauge the climate of different wards; noticeable differences appeared in staff perceptions of their recognition and regard, working relationships, team climate and workload. One ward had high scores for team-working, recognition and regard, and working relationships, coinciding with lower dissatisfaction with workload. This was an admissions ward with very high levels of patient and staff activity. It also boasted earliest and highest compliance with new guidelines, highlighting the significance of local climate for practice development. The approach to test local climate taken in the EBPRAC projects, where 'outsider' project facilitators were working in each care home with mixed groups with little experience of working together, was to use open questions about 'what it's like to work here' as ice-breakers for meetings, and audio-recorded as baseline exploratory data collection strategies.

Implementation strategies need to be planned to match local culture and expectations: How is change usually introduced? Are staff accustomed to being told what to do or are they used to self-determination? Where does the usual managerial approach lie between the extremes of enforced compliance and self-motivated adherence? Redfern et al (2000, p.157) describe one project with a mismatch between a project leader with a personal preference to encourage and motivate working with staff who waited to be enforced because that was what they expected and was the norm in their environment. In this instance, guideline implementation was slow until the project leader matched her approach to local expectations instead of trying to change the staff to meet her ideals.

Information on previous experiences of change in the organisation will be helpful: How have previous changes been handled? How was this viewed by staff? What worked well and what problems were reported? The answers to these questions explained the cynicism encountered in one area in response to attempts to involve staff in project development. A previous communication failure over ward relocation had left staff perceiving a *fait accompli* where managers believed they had consulted and discussed. Efforts to include staff were redoubled rather than rejection being taken at face value.

Further information should include whether anything similar has been tried before, and with what result?

- Some of the staff involved with TKR2 had been involved with an earlier TKR pathway redesign project. This project had big aims and generated big expectations, but failure to deliver had created disillusion.
- Perry et al (2000, p.38) found that a nutrition risk screening tool had been introduced a year before, with little success. However, the two wards which used it wanted to keep it, so it was decided to capitalise on and top up previous training and relaunch the same tool. Whilst improvements in nutrition risk screening were achieved, usage remained poor. It was postulated that rather than building on existing knowledge, relaunch may have been tainted by previous failure.

Similar findings occurred across other projects, leading Redfern et al (2000, p.92) to suggest that it may be easier to generate enthusiasm for something new than to enhance or resurrect existing procedures.

Identifying local stakeholders

The early exploratory phase involves identifying the key players in the topic and for the project, including service users and stakeholders (those with a vested interest in the change). The views of stakeholders and opinion leaders on the envisaged changes should be explored. The TKR2 project leader started the project with a firm belief that psychological elements of pre-operative preparation were the project priority. The physiotherapy representatives saw other priorities. Relationships between individuals' beliefs, attitudes, intentions and behaviours are seldom direct and straightforward. However, while they are poor predictors of behaviour, attitudes clearly influence actions. In discussion with key individuals in advance of a project focused on nutrition support post stroke, it became clear that the risk of inappropriate treatment was a major concern (Perry et al 2000). Decisions about nutritional support for severely disabled patients who are perceived to have poor prognoses can be ethically difficult and compounded by differences of interpretation where future quality of life is the issue. Personal values are also an important contributor to attitudes and actions, a point recognised and explicitly considered within Action Research and Practice Development.

Engaging grassroots workers

Similar considerations argue for investigation of the views of grassroots staff. These are the people who will be asked to enact new ways of working, who will be expected to change their work patterns or activities. One of the key areas to explore is the priority that they accord the topic:

- Care staff in two EBPRAC care homes were unanimous in regarding the meals as a central point in their residents' lives; in seeing provision of each resident with meals that met their needs and preferences as their right; and of the near-impossibility of achieving this with their cook–chill catering system.

- The perceived high priority of cardiovascular health promotion was a key element for a successful Canadian programme (Greenhalgh et al 2004, p.291). Conversely, the low status accorded to some project activities is believed to have hampered knowledge translation, e.g. in the areas of continence (Bignell et al 2000, pp.20, 27) and leg ulcer care (Doherty et al 2000, p.13).

- Low numbers of patients requiring leg ulcer management in individual nurses' caseload restricted ability to practise skills and gain expertise, compounding difficulties in maintaining project activities as a priority (Marshall et al 2001).

Project team members may be best placed to ensure that those healthcare practitioners within their own professional groups are informed of and agree the significance and relevance of the topic. It is also worth exploring the anticipated impact of the practice change upon resourcing and workload patterns. Redfern et al (2000, p.49) note that practitioners in all projects and disciplines reported staff shortages and heavy workloads, a view echoed for the EBPRAC projects (Perry et al 2010a). Doherty et al (2000, p.14) describe a vicious cycle in which lack of time to release community staff nurses for training in leg ulcer management had resulted in a habit of referral to the specialist leg ulcer team. Specialist care effectively decreased community team workload so there was no motivation to release staff for training that would lighten the load on the specialist team but increase it for front-line staff.

Considering users' views

Service users' views are equally important; clients often 'knew jolly well what they wanted from and liked about the service but were not usually asked' (Bignell, personal communication). The priority accorded to the topic by patients themselves is important; healing of leg ulcers was not always a priority for older patients with high levels of co-morbidity and other more pressing problems (Marshall et al 2001). Asking care home residents about mealtimes in the dining room revealed that tensions between the multiple functions of care homes also played out during meals; managing residents' disabilities, health and medication needs could conflict with creation of a homely social ambiance (Moxey et al 2010). Asking about their transition experience as they moved from paediatric to adult services, revealed that young people with type 1 diabetes living in rural areas had a good understanding of the pressures of rural health services, and were all too aware of mismatches between what was available and what they felt would be helpful for their management (Perry et al 2008, Perry et al 2010b).

Identifying possible levers, supports, supporters, hindrances and/or barriers to change

A useful approach to collating all of these elements is the PARiHS framework (Fig. 9.2). Table 9.3 indicates what was found when EBPRAC care homes were assessed for receptiveness for change (this formed one part of the assessment of 'context' for change) using PARiHS. Further detail of the sites and settings was unpacked to get a clearer picture of these sites as environments for change. Interested readers can view this detail in the web version (see Table 9.4 on the website).

Other options include constructing a force field analysis to identify factors expected to promote and support or hinder and resist the endeavour (Lewin 1951) as was done in advance of a practice development within an existing leg ulcer service (Box 9.4; Doherty et al 2000); or carrying out a SWOT analysis to identify potential or actual strengths, weaknesses, opportunities and

TABLE 9.3 'CONTEXT' CHARACTERISTICS THAT INFLUENCED CHANGE IN CARE HOMES: 'RECEPTIVE CONTEXTS' FOR CHANGE

PARiHS variables:	EBPRAC variables
Physical location	Rural and urban settings, but similar staffing issues. Setting characteristics are further unpacked in Table 9.4 available on the web version
Professional networks	Organisational networks – internal monthly meeting
Power and authority	Leadership style
Fit with organisational goals	Nutrition a recognised problem
Skills and knowledge	Varied skills and knowledge of all staff

BOX 9.4 Analysis to identify forces for and against further practice development within an existing leg ulcer service (Doherty et al 2000, with permission)

Forces for change

Open to communication and collaboration

Will accept and cope with small-scale change

Will co-operate if benefit can be seen in the long run

Ground staff eager to gain skills, increase professional development

Enthusiastic teams, young eager staff, negotiation

Senior managerial and trust board support

Desire to have more control over own practice

May perceive relative advantage to change/review practice

Forces against change

Previous bad experience of change in this area

Excessive recent change/low tolerance for change

Increased staff shortage and skills shortage (resource constraint)

Staff shortage and skills shortage (resource constraint)

Management style, viewed as low priority

Staff not motivated to provide this care; 'not interested'

No feedback/incentives; no perceived need for change

New staff not yet fully integrated into trust; may view change as criticism of their standard of care

threats offered by the project as illustrated in Box 9.5, which shows the findings of an analysis carried out in advance of implementing standardised multidisciplinary assessment for older adults prior to hospital discharge (O'Tuathail et al 2000). Both these approaches can serve to focus activities, and as a memory aid as the project progresses. A second example of a force-field analysis (see Table 9.5 on the website) with concise notation of key features supporting and deterring implementation of a valid and reliable swallow screening tool, facilitated planning and tracking of the change process. Choice of approach is a matter for individual nurses; what is important is to ensure that this key phase for any project is not neglected or skimped. Time spent at this point may prevent time wasted later and avoid opposition or distress.

BOX 9.5 SWOT analysis (O'Tuathail et al 2000, with permission)

Strengths
Process to develop care focused on the patient
Opportunity to develop teamwork
Generate multidisciplinary documentation
Create data for audit purposes
Develop evidence-based practice

Weaknesses
Implementation takes time and effort.
May be seen as yet another change.
Yet more paperwork
Large project involving so many disciplines
Large clinical team

Opportunities
Develop better outcomes for patients
Assist trust's contracting process and image of promoting quality care
Marketing initiative regionally and nationally
Improve communication across the primary/secondary interface

Threats
Lack of time for meetings, education sessions and ever-increasing workload
Lack of commitment from individuals or professional groups
Overlap with other ongoing projects
Resistance to change

Knowledge

What evidence is there to defend a course of action other than the status quo? How good is the research? How may it influence the quality of the service as perceived by staff and patients? These are all important questions, the answers to which may have a marked influence on practitioners' and their managers' commitment to the proposed change.

Ensuring change is based on best evidence

A key consideration when setting out to persuade clinicians to alter their behaviours is the quantity and especially the quality of supporting evidence. For many aspects of nursing care, research evidence is limited or incomplete. One important example of this relates to the older elderly (over 85 years), who are often excluded from research studies and, as a result, little information is available to inform us how people in this age group will respond to interventions. Where evidence is lacking, clinical expertise represents 'best available evidence'. If the opinions of local experts are not in tune with recommendations of 'respected authorities', it may be a major challenge to effect changes in practice in the face of resistance factors and the prevailing norms of peer group behaviour. Gaining support for changes underpinned by expert opinion alone if local 'experts' do not endorse it, is likely to be difficult.

Even for those topics where there is strong evidence of advantage for changes in practice, those involved in putting this into place must be persuaded of its relative advantage for themselves and their patients. As a consequence, the project co-ordinator should allow time for discussion and negotiation, and reframing the evidence to the local context (Greenhalgh et al 2004).

Gerrish and Clayton (2004) found that nurses were much more proficient at accessing information such as policies, procedures and guidelines, than research publications, so where resources such as these are developed as part of a service change, or are used within a service, they should reflect current, best evidence. Evidence-based guidelines, discussed in Chapter 7, provide a user-friendly means to communicate research evidence and guidance on 'best practice'. Even in the absence of research evidence there are options to use opinion derived from clinical experience and experts in the field, in the form of consensus statements from working parties, standing committees and conference meetings, often sought using formal methods such as the nominal group process, Delphi technique or consensus development panels (Bowling 1997, pp. 362–365). Auditing of clinical practice against the guideline recommendations may indicate practice development topics.

Other approaches developed to present evidence to healthcare practitioners in brief, user-friendly formats include care pathways, discussed in Chapter 10, which allow incorporation of research evidence into a framework against which the anticipated management and progress of typical patients with specific diagnoses are mapped daily (Wigfield & Boon 1996) and benchmarking, whereby 'best practice' features are identified for local comparison. The latter approach has been taken up in a number of ways; for example, the PACES (Practical Application of Clinical Evidence System) audit framework of the Joanna Briggs Institute (http://paces.jbiconnectplus.org/), the Health Round Table (https://www.healthroundtable.org) and CALNOC, the Collaborative Alliance for Nursing Outcomes (https://www.calnoc.org/globalPages/mainpage.aspx). Additionally, national specialist interest groups conduct national audits, providing data for local benchmarking; for example, the National Sentinel Stroke Audits (http://www.rcplondon.ac.uk/clinical-standards/ceeu/Current-work/stroke/Pages/Audit.aspx).

For both the clinical effectiveness lead initiating a project and the individual nurse seeking help with a practice issue, literature searching and critical appraisal of the evidence identified is a starting point. The chapters in Section 2 address this in detail and this section simply reiterates the importance of (i) making full use of all available resources to track down relevant evidence, including evidence of staff and users' views/patients' perspectives where relevant to that particular service change, (ii) seeking first the most useful types of evidence (such as evidence-based guidelines) rather than individual primary research studies, (iii) assessing the validity and generalisability of the identified evidence and (iv) recognising the usefulness of publications identified; for example, where relevant nationally developed guidelines are identified, it may be sensible to tailor these to suit local circumstances. The 'localising' of nationally developed guidance has been commended by the NHS Executive (1996) and Greenhalgh et al (2004), and may offer the twin benefits of minimising time spent on literature searching and appraisal whilst maximising input of local clinicians to ensure that guidelines address local circumstances and needs.

Intervention

If the proposed service change is small and localised, the nurse may not need a very detailed plan. However, it is always wise to think the process through from all angles before launching into change, and it is essential to ensure that potential implications for any other areas of practice have been considered.

For a large service change it may be beneficial to take a staged approach and address components incrementally. If it is to be introduced across a large area, a rolling programme (perhaps one ward or team at a time) may allow focused intensive input. Identifying one area to function as a 'demonstration project', with systematic evaluation disseminated prior to full roll-out, allows early successes to be seen to be achieved, thus encouraging practitioners and supporting the implementation process. However, incremental implementation may take longer and, although it may achieve better or more sustained response, it may not be feasible within the time available.

Demonstrating baseline practice and the impact of changes

An important element of the change process is the ability to demonstrate whether change has, indeed, occurred and if it has achieved what was expected. With this in mind, before introducing the change in practice, it is useful to carry out a baseline evaluation of current practice both to enable prioritisation of areas of practice where changes are required, and to allow for comparison of practice at a later date via subsequent repetition of the data collection exercise. This is essential if the organisation is to learn what has been gained from this whole process. Consequences of a change in practice may not only occur in intended and predicted areas; there may also be unintentional and unpredictable outcomes ('knock-on' effects) that the organisation may need to address. Evaluation can be a useful 'selling' point for the change management strategy, helping to win support.

Many evidence-based practice change projects are based on existing guidelines with linked audit programmes facilitating collection of data to measure change. National guideline and audit programmes are established for many of the major disease groups (e.g. myocardial infarction and stroke; http://www.rcplondon.ac.uk/clinical-standards/organisation/partnership/Pages/MINAP-.aspx and http://www.rcplondon.ac.uk/clinical-standards/ceeu/Completed-work/Pages/Stroke-audit.aspx). Other processes also entail feedback of information on local outcomes to local clinicians or groups, for example from the National Confidential Enquiries (http://www.ncepod.org.uk/reports.htm), the Intensive Care National Audit & Research Centre (https://www.icnarc.org), and the National Cardiac Arrest Audit (http://www.hqip.org.uk/national-cardiac-arrest-audit-ncaa-2/).

Relevant data to evaluate care processes may be accessible through routinely available data (e.g. pharmacy records may indicate unit usage of naloxone, which may reflect local sedation practices). Patient outcomes (such as pneumonia, pressure sores, falls) may be extracted from routinely collected case mix data or incident monitoring systems. Clinical audit staff are a useful resource for guiding the choice of data. Although much information is routinely collected within organisations, there are often limitations in the manner in which it is presented (e.g. data on length of hospital stay may only be recorded as finished consultant episodes), its detail and accuracy. Where information is not routinely collected, additional effort and resources may be warranted to achieve greater accuracy/relevance, and this is particularly likely to be the case for obtaining users' perspectives.

One angle on patients' and users' views can be gauged through complaints; a broader view may be gained through collecting patient stories. Multiple data collection approaches can be used, and whilst it is beyond the scope of this text to detail these, any good research methods or QI text will do this.

Technical and humanistic elements of change

Changing practice entails two levels of preparation: firstly, the *technical elements*, identifying the practice that needs to change to become aligned with the evidence and what is required to enact this, such as ensuring resources and workflows match new procedures. Secondly, the *humanistic elements*, planning those activities, such as education and training to prepare staff for new ways of working and development and approval of protocols, that will facilitate and enable change. Whilst delivery of information and skills training can ensure that staff are technically able to deliver new services, the ways in which the education and training are delivered can engage staff with the new practices, and predispose them to use their new skills. Humanistic elements of the practice change plan entail using local knowledge to ensure the changes occur as easily and in as problem-free a manner as possible. This latter entails purposefully developing strategies to ensure that:

- support is recruited at all necessary levels of the organisation
- potential barriers and resistance factors are identified and managed
- cultural fit between project and organisational aims and activities is assured
- clinician behaviour aligns with changes to new work processes.

Reviewing implementation studies, Greenhalgh et al (2004, p.292) concluded that many of the factors identified as key to the success and sustainability of changes in practice were highly individual to studies' contexts, and interacted in unique and often unpredictable ways. Hence, a good understanding of the organisational environment and local culture, and service users' views and perspectives is crucial, and identification of the local project manager, sponsors and champions are important steps.

Negotiating roles and responsibilities

Project manager

A primary consideration is the practice development or project manager/leader/co-ordinator role – the person who will hold day-to-day responsibility for the project. Having the right person with the right skills located in the right post within the organisation has been repeatedly identified as crucial for clinical effectiveness/practice development work (Miller et al 1999, Redfern et al 2000, p.155). Miller et al (1999) stress matching the actual post with changes planned; ensuring adequate time, positional and legitimate authority with salary scale reflecting skills and level of responsibility.

Reviewing the range of skills required by the nine STEP1 project managers, Ross and McLaren (2000, p. 25) noted that these spanned communication, research and audit skills, clinical credibility, guideline development and change management experience. The nurse who occupies this position may have worked locally for many years and be well acquainted with the workplace teams, the institution and healthcare locally. However, practice development initiatives are also feasible and appropriate when initiated and/or managed by a nurse new to the area; strengths and limitations attach to both positions. 'Insider' status carries obvious immediate advantages; the nurse knows the system and knows who does what and who to persuade to make things happen. Access to data, personnel and clinical areas may be automatic and clinical credibility with staff has already been established. However, because the nurse is well known, making a role transition or presenting themselves in a different light may not be straightforward. Colleagues may be slow to adapt to changed roles. Doherty et al (2000, pp.14–15) describe difficulties and workload pressures when staff and managers continued to perceive an individual as a clinical nurse specialist despite a role change to practice development. The situation may be complicated where the project lead post is part-time and the post-holder continues to occupy a previous 'insider' role for the remainder of the week. Kilbride et al (2005) commented that this allowed the post-holder to maintain clinical credibility and kept her in touch with grassroots stakeholders in a position that facilitated her influence on changes from the bottom up. However, this position was not always comfortable and there were periods when this 'role duality' led to conflicts due to dual responsibilities, workload issues and staff resentment of her reduced clinical input.

Further, objectivity for organisational analysis and observation of working practices entails extra effort to see past the familiar. This also presents potential for bias where the nurse may be evaluating practice in which they were a key player, and which represents considerable past personal investment. This situation may also pose personal difficulties if colleagues and friends construe evaluation as criticism.

The position of the 'incomer' is the reverse of this. Neither is better; both require awareness of potential problems and ability to capitalise on strengths. It may help if the post-holder is appointed early enough to contribute to project planning (Redfern et al 2000, pp. 141, 166). Supervision or at least a peer support arrangement is important for the post-holder throughout, for debriefing and to maintain focus.

Sponsors and champions

It is important to identify a sponsor, a link person within senior management. This is usually someone with managerial responsibilities who can communicate and connect trust and project aims and strategies, including resource issues. Redfern et al (2000, p. 155) discuss the importance of this role and suggest the optimal choice is someone senior enough to have authority to make decisions and mobilise responses, but junior enough to have time for the project and intimate knowledge of the clinical environment. Their attitude towards the project is important. It is important to consider whether existing influential decision-making groups may impact upon project progress, and if so, who will represent them. For STEP2, Kilbride et al (2005) highlighted the importance of project leads achieving access to and later chairing the medical and managerial Stroke Oversight Committee.

Project champions will also be required. These are the people who will be early adopters and role models of new practices; who will speak up for the project and its objectives in any meeting, and generally work to make the new changed practices work in daily practice, taking every opportunity to present its advantages. Champions may not be formally responsible for the project, but their role entails being proactive to promote its success.

Thought should be given to how supporters of the new ways of working will themselves be supported. The STEP2 project leader struggled with a combination of personal and organisational issues, but fared better once senior support was recruited. A Canadian study of implementation of pressure ulcer guidelines found consistent and ongoing administrative support for the leaders to be critical for success (Clarke et al 2005). The EoC e-PD project found that enthusiasm, initial training and support from a project leader got ward-based facilitators started but when experiences were reviewed, the value of peer support systems for the sustainability of momentum was clear. Project leads and co-ordinators themselves need to be supported and supervised, and such support should be recruited early.

The late planning stage

The project co-ordinator/manager will need to check that:

- realistic goals and time frames have been set
- resources are sufficient. Redfern et al (2000, pp.157, 161) suggest that it may be unreasonable to expect projects to be cost-neutral throughout; it may be more realistic to anticipate some degree of investment that will be recouped later
- the project manager/leader/co-ordinator role is enabled to fulfil required activities
- opportunities have been taken to trial or pilot changes where possible
- interim review points have been identified with flexibility built in to enable changes if necessary in light of progress
- review dates for guideline implementation have been set (and for revision of the guidelines themselves, if developed by the project).

Implementing the change

A range of approaches can be taken (see Greenhalgh et al 2004, pp. 70–120):

Most evidence-based changes entail some form of *educational component*, whether formal (such as case studies, problem-based-learning, workshops, skills training) or informal (such as 1:1 individually-responsive teaching), to inform and prepare clinical staff for their new roles and practices. Reviewing 81 trials of educational meetings, Forsetlund et al (2009) found a median 13.6% improvement in adoption of desired practices. Mixed interactive and didactic education meetings were more effective than either didactic meetings (at 6.9%) or interactive meetings (at 3.0%). Adult education principles indicate that adults learn best when material is perceived as relevant for them and presented/situated within their work context. Hence problem-based learning styles may be particularly useful (Baker 2000). A common misconception is that educational printed materials alone will change practice. Compared to no intervention, printed material alone may have an effect on staff behaviour, but effects are small and the clinical significance uncertain (Farmer et al 2008). Written materials are probably best used in combination with other approaches.

In appealing to clinicians as rational beings, *epidemiological stances* are useful as they focus on the scientific merits of a new course of action in which the overall benefits of new processes for the population of interest have been established. Use of evidence-based guidelines are a common example of this approach, where rigorous processes for systematic search and critiquing of an international evidence base have resulted in scientifically recommended processes for population benefit.

Implementation can also be viewed as the *marketing of a product, information or strategies*; the presentation of the product and the channels of information will be chosen and tailored to maximise appeal to the target audience. Social marketing can also be used, where the focus is not just on the attractiveness and desirability of the product or processes but on the attainment of behavioural goals as a means to achieve specific social benefits with altruistic appeal, e.g. better patient outcomes. The products are promoted on the grounds of what the recipients will get by adopting them, and the social benefit that will accrue.

Social interactionism capitalises on the essential gregariousness of human culture: the influence of fellow practitioners and patients is recognised. Opinion leaders (Doumit et al (2007) demonstrated this approach may improve compliance by 10%), role models, patient pressure, peer support and group norms are all acknowledged agents or resistors of change. Any and all of these can be recruited to attach positive social worth and kudos to the desired practices, and hence enhance local motivation for compliance.

Behavioural approaches to change are underpinned by classical theories of behaviour conditioning, i.e. relying on the influence of specific stimuli before or after the desired actions, for example, audit and feedback (Jamtvedt et al 2006) or reminders tagged to notes or built into software, e.g. for clinic review.

Moving from individual to *organisational approaches*, quality care is seen as dependent upon a cascade of inter-related actions that can be supported or hindered by the structures of the organisation itself. This approach is reflected in attitudes towards adverse incidents which move away from individual fault-finding towards whole-systems approaches (Department of Health 2000b). Whilst the structures of the organisation can imbue a high degree of inertia making change difficult, once change is established they can be recruited to stabilise and sustain the changes.

Each of these approaches offers different avenues and strategies to support and enable evidence-based change. It is not envisaged that any one will meet all requirements; a combination tailored to individual situations and needs is recommended (Greenhalgh et al 2004, pp. 259–260). Information from the 'diagnostic analysis' will be invaluable in guiding the choice of implementation strategies. Irrespective of the scale of change, the key principle is of matching specific strategies to local characteristics and to the culture of the organisation to achieve individual objectives.

Interventions should be accommodated within existing structures where possible. Examples of technical practice change objectives for two projects, and two worked examples are available on the website (Boxes 9.6, 9.7 and 9.8).

Maintaining the project and sustaining the change

Monitoring and evaluating progress

Ward et al (2010, p. 4) discuss the options for KT progress as,

(1) a linear process which involve a stepwise progression between individual elements and an identifiable start and end-point;
(2) a cyclical process where elements are still linked via a stepwise progression, but the process follows a repeating cycle;
(3) a dynamic multidirectional process where individual elements are not linked in a linear fashion, but can occur simultaneously or in different sequences.

The examples they cite indicate the first as the least common experience. It is important to maintain close contact with the progress of planned interventions. Be prepared to make changes if things do not work as expected. For example, ward-based swallow screening sessions were originally planned to take place whenever therapists were on the ward seeing patients. This proved unworkable; activities of therapists, nursing staff and patient needs could not be co-ordinated on an opportunistic basis. A programme of timed appointments was adopted, although it entailed administration time, and this was successful.

Maintain the focus on sustainability. Ways to address this will have been identified from the outset and include use of existing structures and processes and involvement of clinical staff in all aspects. For changes in practice to be sustainable, there must be an effective transfer of activities and responsibilities from the project framework and project manager to normal clinical practice and to front line staff. Whilst it is important that someone takes responsibility to drive dissemination and implementation of practice change, continued reliance upon a single individual weakens the long-term sustainability of the new practices. Withdrawal of the project leader should be planned, possibly around a staged progress of relinquishing responsibilities and adoption by practitioners.

Full incorporation of project activities within normal daily practice may be a lengthy process and it should not be assumed that this will occur naturally. For example, evaluation of a STEP1 project, which initiated substantial changes in stroke management, indicated the need for a named individual to continue championing new practices and to drive service development. A business plan was agreed for appointment of a stroke nurse co-ordinator; however, delayed funding resulted in a 1-year hiatus between departure of the project co-ordinator and appointment to the clinical post. During this time, key components of changed practice were eroded. The 9-month project implementation stage had not been adequate to achieve self-sustainability and further efforts were required.

Once formal evaluation of the changes has occurred ensure that the information is disseminated to everyone involved and give public recognition for the time, energy and commitment of those who made things happen. Consider wider publication of both the processes experienced and results achieved. Changes effected and lessons learned from the EPRAC and STEP 1 projects about practice change in care homes have been widely disseminated. Key points are summarised on the website (Boxes 9.9 and 9.10). What has been learnt about the process of change may be as valuable to colleagues as the effects for patient care. Avenues to disseminate findings include local and national conferences, fora and interest group meetings, papers and publications ranging from major international journals to society newsletters. Consumer groups will likely also be interested.

Summary

This chapter has sought to illustrate how evidence-based service changes have been applied within real-life projects. Examples have been drawn from a range of implementation and evaluation projects to demonstrate things which worked and pitfalls to avoid. It would be misleading to suggest that following the processes detailed will guarantee success; changing practice is never easy and no two situations are identical. However, in the world of knowledge transfer there is an increasing wealth of experience to draw on, and outcomes of the projects described in this chapter demonstrate that efforts to implement practice that is explicitly evidence based can be well rewarded.

Exercise

We encourage you to undertake the critical appraisal exercise on the website.

References

ACHCEW (Association for Community Health Councils for England and Wales), 1997. Hungry in hospital? ACHCEW, London.

Baker, C.M., 2000. Problem-based learning for nursing: integrating lessons from other disciplines with nursing experiences. J. Prof. Nurs. 16 (5), 258–266.

Benner, P., 1984. From novice to expert. Addison-Wesley, Menlo Park.

Bignell, V., Getliffe, K., Forester, L., 2000. The South Thames Evidence-based Practice Project. The promotion of continence for elderly people in primary care: the role of community nurses. St George's Hospital Medical School and Kingston University, London.

Bonis, S.A., 2009. Knowing in nursing: A concept analysis. J. Adv. Nurs. 65 (6), 1328–1341.

Bowling, A., 1997. Research methods in health. Open University Press, Buckingham.

Carper, B.A., 1978. Fundamental patterns of knowing in nursing. Adv. Nurs. Sci. 1 (1), 13–23.

Clarke, H.F., Bradley, C., Whytock, S., et al., 2005. Pressure ulcers: implementation of evidence-based nursing practice. J. Adv. Nurs. 49 (6), 578–590.

Clarke, T., Kelleher, M., Fairbrother, G., 2010. Starting a care improvement journey: focusing on the essentials of bedside nursing care in an Australian teaching hospital. J. Clin. Nurs. 19, 1812–1820.

Department of Health, 2000a. An organisation with a memory: report of an expert group on learning from adverse events in the NHS. Available online at www.dh.gov.uk/ assetRoot/04/08/89/48/04088948.pdf (accessed 10.09.05).

Department of Health, 2000b. Research and development for a first class service. R & D funding in the new NHS. Department of Health, Leeds.

Doherty, D., Ross, F., Yeo, L., et al., 2000. The South Thames Evidence-based Practice Project. Leg ulcer management in an integrated service. St George's Hospital Medical School and Kingston University, London.

Doumit, G., Gattellari, M., Grimshaw, J., O'Brien, M.A., 2007. Local opinion leaders: effects on professional practice and health care outcomes. Cochrane Database Syst. Rev. 2007 (1) Art. No.: CD000125. doi:10.1002/14651858.CD000125.pub3.

Farmer, A.P., Légaré, F., Turcot, L., Grimshaw, J., Harvey, E., McGowan, J.L., et al., 2008. Printed educational materials: effects on professional practice and health care outcomes. Cochrane Database Syst. Rev. 2008 (3) Art. No.: CD004398. doi:10.1002/14651858.CD004398.pub2.

Forsetlund, L., Bjørndal, A., Rashidian, A., et al., 2009. Continuing education meetings and workshops: effects on professional practice and health care outcomes. Cochrane Database Syst. Rev. 2009 (2) Art. No.: CD003030. doi:10.1002/14651858.CD003030.pub2.

Gerrish, K., Clayton, J., 2004. Promoting evidence-based practice: an organisational approach. J. Nurs. Manag. 12, 114–123.

Greenhalgh, T., Robert, G., Bate, P., et al., 2004. How to spread good ideas. A systematic review of the literature on diffusion, dissemination and sustainability of innovations in health service delivery and organisation. In: Report for the National Co-ordinating Centre for NHS Service Delivery and Organisation R & D (NCCSDO). Available online at www. sdo.lshtm.ac.uk/pdf/changemanagement_greenhalgh_report.pdf (accessed 10.09.05).

Hart, E., Bond, M., 1995. Action Research for Health and Social Care. Open University Press, Buckingham.

Jamtvedt, G., Young, J.M., Kristoffersen, D.T., O'Brien, M.A., Oxman, A.D., 2006. Audit and feedback: effects on professional practice and health care outcomes. Cochrane Database Syst. Rev. 2006 (2) Art. No.: CD000259. doi:10.1002/14651858. CD000259.pub2.

Kajermo, K.N., Boström, A.-M., Thompson, D.S., et al., 2010. The BARRIERS Scale - the barriers to research utilization scale: A systematic review. Implementation Science 5, 32. Available online at http://www.implementationscience.com/content/5/1/32. Accessed 21 March 2011.

Kilbride, C., Meyer, J., Flatley, M., et al., 2005. Stroke units: the implementation of a complex intervention. Education Action Research 13 (4), 479.

Kilbride, C., Perry, L., Flatley, M., et al., 2010. Developing theory and practice: creation of a Community of Practice through Action Research produced excellence in stroke care. J. Interprof. Care Early Online. 1–8. doi:10.3109/13561820.2010.483024.

Kohn, L.T., Corrigan, J.M., Donaldson, M.S. (Eds.), 1999. To Err Is Human. Building a Safer Health System. Committee on Quality of Health Care in America.

Lewin, K., 1951. Field theory in social science. Harper, New York.

Lister, S., Brodie, L., 2008. Transition Care Workforce Project: Final report. Greater Metropolitan Clinical Taskforce Transition Care Network, Sydney. Available online at http://www.health.nsw.gov.au/resources/gmct/transition/pdf/transition_care_workforce:report.pdf (accessed 08 08 10).

Lucas, B., 2008. Total hip and total knee replacement: preoperative nursing management. Br. J. Nurs. 17 (21), 1346–1351.

Mantzoukas, S., Jasper, M., 2007. Types of nursing knowledge used to guide care of hospitalized patients. J. Adv. Nurs. 62 (3), 318–326.

Marshall, J.L., Mead, P., Jones, K., et al., 2001. The implementation of venous leg ulcer guidelines: process analysis of the intervention used in a multi-centre, pragmatic, randomised, controlled trial. J. Clin. Nurs. 10 (6), 758–766.

McCormack, B., Manley, K., Kitson, A., et al., 1999. Towards practice development—a vision in reality or a reality without vision? J. Nurs. Manag. 7, 255–264.

McCormack, B., Wright, J., Dewar, B., et al., 2007a. A realist synthesis of evidence relating to practice development: Methodology and methods. Practice Development in Health Care 6 (1), 5–24. doi:10.1002/pdh.210.

McCormack, B., Wright, J., Dewar, B., et al., 2007b. A realist synthesis of evidence relating to practice development: Findings from the literature analysis. Practice Development in Health Care 6 (1), 25–55. doi: 10.1002/pdh.211.

Meyer, J., 2000. Evaluating action research. Age Ageing 29, S2 8–10.

Miller, C., Scholes, J., Freeman, P., 1999. Evaluation of the 'assisting clinical effectiveness' programme. In: Humphris, D., Littlejohns, P. (Eds.), Implementing clinical guidelines. A practical guide. Radcliffe Press, Oxford.

Moxey, A., Byles, J., Perry, L., et al., 2010. Residents' perspectives on the meals and dining experience in residential aged care. Australian Association of Gerontology Rural Conference, April 2010, Ballina.

NHS Executive, 1996. Clinical guidelines. Using clinical guidelines to improve patient care within the NHS. NHS Executive, Leeds.

Nolan, M., Grant, G., Brown, J., et al., 1998. Assessing nurses' work environment: old dilemmas, new solutions. Clinical Effectiveness in Nursing 2, 145–156.

NSW Dept of Health Nursing and Midwifery Office, 2009. Working with Essentials of Care: a resource guide for facilitators. Sydney.

O'Tuathail, C., Ross, F., Stubberfield, D., 2000. The South Thames Evidence-based Practice Project. Standardised multidisciplinary assessment of older people on discharge from hospital. St George's Hospital Medical School and Kingston University, London.

Perry, L., McLaren, S., 2000. An evaluation of implementation of evidence-based guidelines for dysphagia screening and assessment following acute stroke: phase 2 of an evidence-based practice project. Journal of Clinical Excellence 2, 147–156.

Perry, L., McLaren, S., Bennett, M., 2000. The South Thames Evidence-based Practice Project. Nutritional support for patients with acute stroke. St George's Hospital Medical School and Kingston University, London.

Perry, L., Lowe, J., Steinbeck, K., et al., 2008. What makes a quality service for a 'hard to access' group in rural locations? Users' views of services for young people with Type 1 diabetes in rural New South Wales. Royal College of Nursing Research Society Conference, April 2008, Cardiff, Wales.

Perry, L., Bellchambers, H., Howie, A., et al., 2011. Does the PARIHS framework 'work' for aged care? Examining the utility of a framework for implementation of evidence based practice in residential aged care settings. In press J. Adv. Nurs.

Perry, L., Steinbeck, K.S., Dunbabin, J., et al., 2010b. Lost in transition? Access, uptake and outcomes of services for young people with Type 1 diabetes in regional New South Wales. Accepted by Med. J. Aust. June 2010.

Porter, S., O'Halloran, P., 2008. The postmodernist war on evidence-based practice. Int. J. Nurs. Stud. 46, 740–749.

Redfern, S., Christian, S., Murrells, T., et al., 2000. Evaluation of change in practice: South Thames Evidence-based Practice Project (STEP). King's College, London.

Ross, F., McLaren, S., 2000. The South Thames Evidence-based Practice Project. An overview of aims, methods and cross-case analysis of nine implementation projects. St George's Hospital Medical School and Kingston University, London.

Rycroft-Malone, J., Kitson, A., Harvey, G., et al., 2002. Ingredients for change: revisiting a conceptual framework. Qual. Health Care 11 (2), 174–180.

Special Commission of Inquiry, Garling, P. (Chair), 2008. Acute Care in NSW Public Hospitals, 2008. Available online at http://www.lawlink.nsw.gov.au/acsinquiry. Accessed 21 March 2011.

Spenceley, S.M., O'Leary, D.A., Chizawsky, L., et al., 2008. Sources of information used by nurses to inform practice: An integrative review. Int. J. Nurs. Stud. 45, 954–970.

Straus, S.E., Tetroe, J., Graham, I., 2009. Defining knowledge translation. Can. Med. Assoc. J. 181 (34), 165–168.

Tanner, C., 2006. Thinking like a nurse: a research-based model of clinical judgment in nursing. J. Nurs. Educ. 45 (6), 204–211.

Thompson, C., 2003. Clinical experience as evidence in evidence-based practice. J. Adv. Nurs. 43 (3), 230–237.

Thompson, C., Cullum, N., McCaughan, D., et al., 2004. Nurses, information use, and clinical decision making — the real world potential for evidence-based decisions in nursing. Evid. Based Nurs. 7, 68–72.

Ward, V., Smith, S., Carruthers, S., et al., 2010. Knowledge Brokering. Exploring the process of transferring knowledge into action. Final Report. University of Leeds, UK.

Waterman, H., Tillen, D., Dickson, R., et al., 2001. Action research: a systematic review and guidance for assessment. Health Technol. Assess. 2001 (5), 23. Availabe online at http://www.hta.ac.uk/project/1007.asp. (accessed 18.10.10).

Westwood, N., James-Moore, M., Cooke, M., 2007. Going Lean in the NHS. NHS Institute for Innovation and Improvement. At http://www.institute.nhs.uk/option,com_joomcart/Itemid,26/main_page,document_product_info/products_id,231.html. Accessed 21 March 2011.

Wigfield, A., Boon, E., 1996. Critical care pathway development: the way forward. Br. J. Nurs. 5 (12), 732–735.

10
CHAPTER

How can we develop an evidence-based culture?

Carl Thompson

KEY POINTS

- Evidence-based change is a national policy imperative and unavoidable in practice.
- Evidence-based culture is one which is totally committed to balanced decisions that give due weight to research evidence, patient preference, available resources and clinical expertise. This commitment is manifest at the levels of the individual, clinical teams and healthcare systems.
- Successful strategies for change are likely to be multifaceted and targeted at specific cultural groups in the organisation.
- Specific groups for targeted and planned change interventions are best identified through sensitive diagnostic strategies.

- Theoretical models such as social marketing may prove useful as a way of structuring change strategies, but evidence to date is lacking.

- Consistently effective interventions include educational outreach, electronic or paper-based reminders and multifaceted approaches.

- Audit and feedback alone has a mixed and unpredictable impact on changing professional behaviour and culture.

- Didactic study days, clinical guidelines and protocols that are passively disseminated have little or no effect on practice.

Introduction

Culture shapes the beliefs and behaviours of those who deliver health care. Without an awareness of the impact of culture on the utilisation of research evidence, strategies for change will almost certainly fail. However, cultural change is hard to achieve in ways that are simple to predict (Davies et al 2000, Parker 2000, Scott et al 2003). Real-world, realistic strategies for evidence-based change in organisations require well-planned, targeted, informed strategies that incorporate what we know about both culture and the foreseeable effects of general and specific change interventions. Organisations such as the UK's NHS Service Delivery and Organisation Research and Development Programme (NHS SDO) and the Veteran's Administration (VA) and Agency for Healthcare Research and Quality (AHRQ) in the USA have funded research and development that has extended our empirical and theoretical knowledge considerably since previous editions of this book. This chapter aims to steer a course through some of these developments.

National imperatives

A greater role for knowledge derived from scientific research in improving the quality of health services is a policy objective for almost all developed countries. Using the UK as an exemplar, since the late 1990s, the UK government has pursued a systematic approach to quality improvement in the National Health Service (NHS). Clinical governance (Secretary of State for Health 1998) is the term intended to encapsulate this approach: 'A framework through which NHS organisations are accountable for continuously improving the quality of their services and safeguarding high standards of care by creating an environment in which excellence in clinical care will flourish' (p. 33). The evolution of a model of service commissioning and provision in the UK NHS means that the managers and clinicians who purchase services on behalf of communities are also expected to use research to inform these decisions (Department of Health 2007).

The boards of NHS organisations now have a formal duty to ensure that quality is improved, and bodies such as the National Institute for Health and Clinical Excellence (NICE), National Service Frameworks (NSF), and the Health-Care Commission, have been established to assist this process. Chief Executives, who are subject to audit of the overall performance of their organisations (Secretary of State for Health 2000), are increasingly scrutinising the quality of healthcare provision in individual clinical areas. In the United States, the Agency for Healthcare Research and Quality (AHRQ), a federal sub-agency of the Department of Health and Human Services, has, since the late 1990s, explicitly fostered evidence-based provision of health care through a range of evaluative initiatives in key areas. Examples of such initiatives include the use of information technology to improve health and reducing disparities between communities. Individual professional groups are similarly experiencing a policy 'push' towards evidence-based decision-making. Individual employer organisations and the nursing profession itself are firmly committed to addressing the difficult task of aligning quality, knowledge and the action of practitioners, so the question 'How can we best develop an evidence-based practice culture?' looks more relevant than ever.

What does an evidence-based culture look like?

Organisational culture: what is it?

Culture is a contested concept. Despite the many ways of conceptualising it, two discernible strands emerge: culture as something that an organisation *is*, but also something that an organisation *has,* in the form of attributes or variables that can be identified and shaped (Davies et al 2000). This distinction is important, for if organisations are the products of culture then there is considerably less scope for manipulating and shaping progress towards organisational goals. On the other hand, if organisations *have* culture – if they possess attributes and values – then shaping and actively managing culture in order to reinforce strategic aims and goals becomes a possibility. Davies and colleagues (2000) suggest 10 key aspects of organisational culture (Box 10.1) that may be the focus of

---

BOX 10.1 Ten key features of organisational culture (adapted from Davies et al 2000)

Attitudes to innovation and risk taking: the degree to which the organisation encourages and rewards new ways of doing things or, conversely, values tradition

Degree of central direction: the extent of central setting of objectives and performance versus devolved decision-making

Patterns of communication: the degree to which instruction and reporting are channelled via formal hierarchies rather than informal networks

Outcome or process orientation: whether the organisation values (focuses on) outcomes and results as opposed to tasks

Internal or external focus: whether the organisation looks inward and restricts itself to organisational issues as opposed to looking at the needs of customers

Uniformity or diversity: the organisational propensity towards consistency or diversity

People orientation: valuation of the human resources available to an organisation

Team orientation: does the organisation reward individualism or is it geared more towards teamwork?

Aggressiveness/competitiveness: the extent to which the organisation seeks to dominate or cooperate with external competitors or players

Attitudes to change: the extent to which the organisation demonstrates a predilection for stability in preference to dynamic change

management efforts to align an organisation towards its strategic aims; strategic aims such as the provision of increasingly evidence-based decisions as a route to better quality patient care.

An evidence-based practice culture

Muir Gray (1997) suggests that the basis for healthcare provision is the decisions made within its structures and organisations. An evidence-based practice culture is one in which more good decisions are made than bad, and where research evidence, patient preferences, the available resources and clinical expertise play an active part in decision-making processes (DiCenso et al 1998, Sackett et al 2000) (Fig. 10.1).

The key components of an evidence-based organisation, then, are:

> *a built-in ... capability to generate, and the flexibility to incorporate, evidence and individuals and teams who can find, appraise and use research evidence (Muir Gray 1997, p. 155).*

In order to achieve these characteristics, the organisation is dependent on the cultures, systems and structures contained

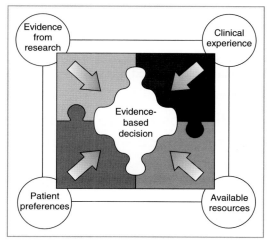

Figure 10.1 An evidence-based healthcare decision

within it. Moreover, all these elements share a degree of inter-dependence; systems that promote evidence-based decisions are no use unless accompanied by supportive structures and a facilitative cultural environment.

Evidence-based health care has five key processes:

1. Converting healthcare problems into focused health-care questions
2. Searching for the best available research evidence
3. Critically appraising the evidence retrieved
4. Implementing the evidence
5. Auditing the implementation.

Evidence-based organisational culture is one in which individuals and groups are totally committed to each of these stages and at all organisational levels. Brown (1999) notes that an organisational culture for evidence-based health care requires commitment at the level of:

- the individual
- clinical teams or practice groups
- healthcare systems and organisations.

Before embarking on any attempt to change the culture of an organisation or group, key questions need addressing (Illes & Sutherland 2001), the most important of which is establishing why change is required and who and what can change. Only when this vital element of context has been mapped is it possible to plan for change.

Step one: diagnosing the challenges to changing practice – understanding complexity

Because changing cultures is complex, it is necessary to spend time trying to understand this complexity. In order to make sense of the context surrounding any planned change, a number of frameworks are available to help the manager or nurse. These include the 7s model, soft systems methodology, content context and process modelling and the '5 Whys' approaches (Illes & Sutherland 2001). These approaches vary in the effort and scope required to put them into practice. Accordingly, readers who require more detail of the methods are encouraged to look at the review by Illes and Sutherland (www.sdo.lshtm.ac.uk/pdf/changemanagement_ review.pdf). However, some of the techniques are relatively simple to operationalise. For example, the '5 Whys' approach involves simply asking the question 'why?' of a situation in which the focus is a single problem (see Box 10.2).

Any approach chosen as the basis for making sense of the complexity of a situation should:

- identify all the groups involved in, affected by or influencing the proposed change(s) in practice
- assess the characteristics of the proposed change that might influence its adoption
- assess the preparedness of health professionals to change and other potentially relevant internal factors within the target group

---

BOX 10.2 The '5 whys' approach to understanding complexity

Problem: nurses are routinely ordering (unnecessary) urine tests on children who do not require them.

Why does this happen? It is seen as a necessary routine part of admission screening.

Why? Nurses do not understand the clinical value of looking at signs and symptoms and prevalence alongside the 'dipstick' urinalysis test they undertake.

Why? Nurses do not know about the positive predictive value of a test such as urinalysis.

Why? Nurses do not know what positive predictive value means and how to estimate it 'on the fly' in routine practice.

Why? Because they have not been introduced to the concept in practice and had its application reinforced.

- identify the potential external barriers to change
- identify the likely enabling factors, including resources and skills (NHS CRD 1999).

Whilst these approaches are useful frameworks, they require gathering data as the means of providing answers to the questions generated. Techniques to consider as means of generating these data include:

- surveying key stakeholders (such as senior staff, managers and patient representatives) to identify the research appraisal and change management skills available. Similarly, some of the perceived barriers to research utilisation could be explored using survey approaches such as Funk's 'Barriers' Scale (Funk et al 1991). It is important to recognise, however, that reported barriers to utilisation may only capture those dimensions that individuals feel comfortable revealing. Moreover, in the field of research utilisation, what people say they do and what they actually do are often separate (Covell et al 1985, McCaughan et al 2005). The diagnostic value of this tool has not been established and so it is probably best considered as part of a broader suite of diagnostic activity
- adapting ward meetings or clinical supervision sessions so that potential problems can be identified, recorded and fed into the strategic planning process
- establishing focus groups of professionals, managers and, where appropriate, patients or their representatives, to identify pertinent barriers and drivers. Cameron & Wren (1999) used this approach by forming 'buzz' groups of 6–8 people who used 'reflection-on-action' (Schon 1983) to identify their values. These were typed and distributed to the group who then worked towards a collective understanding of the values identified.

Step two: how can evidence-based innovation and culture be encouraged?

Evidence-based innovation includes those new behaviours, routines and ways of working that are intended to improve health outcomes (Greenhalgh et al 2004). These innovations rarely happen by themselves; rather, they are planned and deliberate. Whilst there is no magic formula (Oxman et al 1995) for developing innovations, much is known about the ingredients required, even if the optimal 'mixes' remain hidden.

There are three major dimensions that must be addressed by anyone considering cultural change – to the point where it is manifest as changes in behaviour:

- The innovation itself
- The individuals and groups involved
- The system in which the innovation must operate.

Because none of the three elements operates in isolation from the others it is useful to add a fourth dimension to this list:

- The linkages (between the innovation, its systemic context and the individuals involved).

The innovation

Those characteristics of the innovation itself associated with positive uptake in organisations are highlighted in Box 10.3.

The individual

Individuals work creatively with their organisations, and the individual differences that mark out team members also extend to the ways in which they interact with innovations. In order to maximise the chances of change adoption by a team and its members, it is important to understand some key characteristics in the individual, team or work unit involved. Box 10.4 summarises the key dimensions to be charted.

The organisation as a knowledge-driven system

Using management to develop an organisation's structural and cultural components is a necessary step in encouraging assimilation of evidence-based innovations. The structural components

---

BOX 10.3 Attributes of an innovation associated with adoption

Standard or universal attributes	Operational or context-specific attributes
Relative advantage: the degree to which a clear and unambiguous effectiveness or cost-effectiveness beyond 'where we are now' is present. Remembering that 'advantage' is often constructed by negotiations between stakeholders	*Innovation:* has to be seen as relevant for the adopter's work tasks
Compatibility: fit with the values and norms of the workplace	*Performance improving*: an innovation should be seen to improve performance in a given task
Complexity: simple (or the ability to break down the innovation into a simple form) equates with higher chances	*Perceived feasibility*: in a given context
Trialability: can the innovation be tried out and experimented within the workplace?	*Divisibility*: the ability to break it down into manageable components
Observability: observable benefits increase adoption	*Codified and transferable know ledge*: the degree to which the knowledge needed to actually make use of the innovation can be separated from one context and transferred to another
Reinvention: the ability to shape an innovation to suit one's own needs equates to a higher chance of adoption	

---

of an organisation and their relationship to innovativeness (a key component of an evidence-based culture) are summarised in Table 10.1.

As can be seen from Table 10.1, a number of elements of culture can be manipulated in an organisation's drive to foster innovation. Not all the elements of an organisational system are within the direct control of a clinician or individual manager; they are, however, important elements of context to be borne in mind when developing change strategies.

BOX 10.4 Considerations at the level of the individual

Psychological precursors: cognitive and social psychology literature suggests that the degree to which someone is tolerant of ambiguity, their intellect and their general values towards change will influence their propensity for trying new ideas. If the individual has identified a need and the innovation meets that need then change is more likely.

Meaning: the meaning that an innovation may have for an adopter needs to be established. If this meaning fits the meaning associated with management and other stakeholding groups then adopting an innovation is more likely.

Adoption decision nature: is the decision to opt into the innovation contingent (i.e. does it depend on someone else in the organisation?) or authoritative (a compulsory activity). Whilst authoritative decisions may appear to increase chances of initial adoption, they also reduce the chances of long-term adoption.

Adoption decision stage concerns: it is important to remember that adoption is a process rather than a single event. Different concerns arise at different points in this process:

- Before adoption – individuals need to be aware of the pending change and be given enough information to decide how it will affect them.
- During the early stages – training and support to a level which will enable individuals to shape the change to their own working practices must be provided.
- Once the change is established – feedback of the consequences enable individuals to continue to refine the innovation for their own environments.

Another important antecedent for developing an evidence-based culture at the level of systems is the organisation's capacity for absorbing new knowledge. Knowledge in service organisations underpins action; and the degree to which an organisation can codify what it does, capture new information, place it in the organisational context (so that it then becomes knowledge) and then design it into its work practices and decision-making machinery is an important determinant of the service that the public eventually receives (Ferlie et al 2001).

TABLE 10.1 ORGANISATIONAL SYSTEMIC CHARACTERISTICS AND
RELATIONSHIP WITH INNOVATIVENESS IN ORGANISATIONS

Characteristic	Definition	Direction (positive or negative)
Administrative intensity	Administrative costs	+
Centralisation	Autonomy in decision making	–
Complexity	Degrees of profession-alism and specialisation	+
External communication	Extent of workers' participation in professional activity outside the organisation	+
Formalisation	Degree of rule follow-ing and procedures	No significant relationship
Functional differentiation	Number of different work units	+
Internal communication	Communication between units	+
Managerial attitude to change		+
Managers' experience		No significant relationship
Professionalism	Degree of professional knowledge in the organisation	+
'Slackness'	The resources in an organisation that go beyond the minimum required to do the job	+
Specialisation	Number of specialties	+
Technical capacity	Amount of technical resource	+
Hierarchical levels	How many levels there are in the organisation	No significant relationship

The knowledge that shapes social action, provides feedback on performance and 'feed-forward' (or task guidance), is socially constructed in health care. For example, a particular drug may objectively be 'effective', but the integration of patient values, its link to available resources and the expertise of the person delivering it all vary from context to context and, often, is negotiable. Once the contested nature of the knowledge required for managing decisions in health care, what Sackett and others (2000) term 'foreground' knowledge, is acknowledged, then the importance of the science of communication, knowledge management and transfer becomes apparent. As Greenhalgh and colleagues (2004, p. 607) put it:

> ...before it [knowledge] can contribute to organisational change initiatives, knowledge must be enacted and made social, entering into the stock of knowledge constructed and shared by other individuals. Knowledge depends for its circulation on interpersonal networks and will spread only when these social factors and barriers are overcome.

Introducing new knowledge into an environment which is not receptive to change (or the possibility of it) is likely to lead to failure to innovate or change values, motivations and ultimately practice. Greenhalgh and colleagues (2004) suggest a number of indicators of receptive environments: strong leadership skills; clear strategic vision accompanied by managerial relations that help support that vision; key staff with a sense of shared vision; a risk-taking environment where trialling ideas is supported; and good systems of data capture. This last point is an essential component: data form the basis of information which, through the addition of context, then becomes knowledge.

Step three: how can change happen?

Developing an evidence-based change toolkit

Thus far, I have concentrated on outlining some important components of what might be termed a framework for thinking about complexity and innovation in healthcare settings. Considering these components is a necessary step for thinking about cultural change – not least in order to form a contextual backdrop for any planned action. Whilst all these elements are controllable to a greater or lesser degree, it is the level of specific change interventions (or, more accurately, combinations of specific change interventions) that provides the most fertile ground for most nurses to think about changing behaviour and impacting of values and goals relating to healthcare provision.

The previous sections were aimed at diagnosing the change problem, mapping the antecedents of that problem most amenable to intervention, approaching the implementation of change in a planned and systematic way, and considering ways of evaluating its impact. A good start point for this generic approach to managing change generally is the *Clinical Effectiveness: What It's All About* resource pack for nurses and health-care professionals produced by the NHS Executive (1999). Similarly the NHS Service Delivery and Organisation Programme produces a range of publications designed to aid change managers, details of which are presented at the end of the chapter. Whilst these publications are primarily aimed at UK health professionals and managers, they can easily be adapted to a US, Canadian or Australian context.

There is a surprising volume of material that summarises what we know about changing behaviour and managing the transition from abstract research knowledge into improved, and research-informed, professional decisions. Much of the high-quality material derived from randomised controlled trials has been summarised by the Cochrane Collaboration's Effective Practice and Organisation of Care Group (http://epoc.cochrane.org/). Before considering specific elements of a change strategy, it is worth taking the time to think about the nature of the information used as the basis for day-to-day change and how this can be quality assured and the return for the time invested maximised.

Developing evidence-based ward literature: systems, synopses, syntheses and studies

The need to develop a store of good-quality information at ward or unit level arises out of a general recognition that nurses have limited time available for consulting written sources of information and that many resources are out of date and not evidence based. Moreover, obtaining a clinical bottom line for the patient in front of you is often difficult and involves the translation of hard-to-interpret research findings. Many sources are poorly organised, with few individuals being able to rapidly lay their hands on useful written information for every clinical problem. Moreover, nurses often invest time and considerable amounts of money in compiling these inadequate resources. Because of these human traits, wherever possible, change should be supported by a good-quality decision support system. Such systems are rare in nursing, but they do exist, for example in anticoagulation clinics and in primary care in the form of NHS Clinical Knowledge Summaries (http://cks.nhs.uk/home). Where such systems exist, they have the advantage of tailoring research-based clinical knowledge to the uncertainties associated with individual patients.

Where decision support systems do not exist, another efficient means of getting high-quality research messages, with the minimum of effort and maximum applicability, is in the form of synopses. The best forms of accessing synopses of information are the various evidence-based journals (such as *Evidence-based Nursing* and *Evidence-based Medicine*). An alternative that can be used for interventions other than simple pharmaceutical options is Clinical Evidence (www.clinicalevidence.com). These resources have the advantage that the critical appraisal and quality assurance are done for you (saving you time), with 'context' injected by virtue of the accompanying clinical commentary in the evidence-based journals.

Syntheses in the form of systematic reviews offer summarised information, but have the relative disadvantage of requiring critical appraisal. Finally, searching for individual studies, even using computerised technology, is labour intensive, relatively ineffective and uses up scarce time.

Other chapters in this book deal with searching for resources, but the 6S approach to setting up an information strategy, expanded from Brian Haynes' (2001) original 5S approach (DiCenso et al 2009; Fig. 3.4 in Chapter 3, page 65), should be the starting point for anyone seeking to use information to support clinical change.

As healthcare providers embrace electronic information technology (through, for example, NHSNet, and NHS Evidence), it is crucial that nurses acquire the skills to handle information effectively. There is no shortcut available to learning the computer skills needed to use a personal referencing system or online database, but the investment will pay dividends. A first port of call for nurses employed by the NHS or by academic institutions within the UK is the NHS Evidence (http://www.evidence.nhs.uk/), this provides an invaluable source of quality-assured information including links to many of the resources listed below.

What works and what doesn't?

Empirical scrutiny of what works in terms of the behavioural element of getting evidence into practice has led to some tentative estimates of the 'effect size' of various strategies for changing practice and impacting on culture. These effect sizes are sobering. It is clear that the likely gains in performance based on what we know about changing practice may be far lower, and with greater variability, than is often assumed by those developing interventions. Moreover, it appears unlikely that simply combining interventions in the hope that more will be necessarily better exerts a greater or more predictable improvement in performance or its cultural component.

Continuing education: 'study days'

Study days, professional development courses, conference attendance and post registration courses are all common features of many nurses' career trajectories and plans. However, as a stand-alone intervention, study days are not particularly effective. Five systematic reviews (Beaudry 1989, Bertram & Brooks-Bertram 1977, Davis et al 1995, Lloyd & Abrahamson 1979, Waddell 1991) all examine the impact of educational approaches to changing healthcare professional behaviours. Waddell (1991) focuses specifically on nurses. The results are contradictory, with most reviews reporting at least some effect, but the validity of the reviews is hampered by the poor quality of many of the primary research reports. It is significant, however, that the high-quality systematic reviews (Davis et al 1995) conclude that continuing educational approaches are a relatively ineffective way of changing practice. Conversely, those reviews of lesser quality tend towards viewing study days as more effective (Waddell 1991). Grimshaw et al (2004) reported a 1% absolute improvement in performance attributable to educational meetings.

Clinical guidelines

Clinical guidelines have proved an influential and attractive mechanism for influencing behaviour in nursing, with the Royal College of Nursing in the UK committed to sponsoring, and cooperating in, their production. However, as in the case of continuing professional development, their success should not be assumed uncritically. Thomas et al (1999) have undertaken a systematic review of the role of clinical guidelines as a route to reducing inappropriate variations in practice and promoting the delivery of evidence-based health care. They suggest that the best advice for a nurse wishing to use guidelines to change practice is to learn from the experiences of other groups – notably medicine – and to develop strategies that draw on evidence-based theoretical perspectives (Grol 1992). The NHS CRD (1999) found that properly developed guidelines can influence practice, but work best if they are adapted to local circumstance, are used in conjunction with supportive educational strategies and include specific reminders to help professionals in their decision-making.

Some strategies such as integrated care pathways (ICPs) manage to combine at least some of these elements. Pathways are commonly based around local systems and processes, supported by clinical and managerial teams, based on a guideline format and have reminders built into documentation and monitoring technologies which are often part of larger scale clinical audit. The label 'integrated care pathways' contains a heterogeneous combination of interventions; something not lost on those who have sought to systematically review the evidence for their use (Allen et al 2009). Whilst summarizing the results of such disparate meta analyses makes no sense at all, some general conclusions can be offered based on a narrative overview of the studies (Allen et al 2009). First, in relation to 'what works and when':

- In the context of (relatively) predictable trajectories of care ICPs can be effective in supporting proactive care management and ensuring that patients receive relevant and timely clinical interventions and/or assessments.
- ICPs help promote adherence to guidelines or treatment protocols thereby reducing variation in practice.
- ICPs help improve documentation of treatment goals and documentation of communication between patients, carers and health professionals.
- ICPs can be effective in improving physician agreement about treatment options.
- ICPs that contain a decision aid can be effective in supporting decision-making.
- ICPs may be particularly effective in changing professional behaviours in the desired direction, where there is scope for improvement or where roles are new.

Perhaps just as importantly Allen and colleagues also highlight those circumstances in which ICPs are less successful:

- ICPs do not always bring about service quality and efficiency gains in patient trajectories.
- ICPs may be less effective in bringing about quality improvements in circumstances in which services are already based on best evidence and multidisciplinary working is well-established.
- Depending on their purpose, the benefits of ICPs may be greater for certain patient sub-groups than others.
- ICPs may not be cost effective; perhaps because supporting mechanisms to underpin their implementation are needed, particularly in circumstances in which ICP use is a significant change in organisational culture.
- ICP documentation can introduce scope for new kinds of error.

Other broad approaches

A number of systematic reviews examine the effectiveness of broad dissemination and implementation strategies (Oxman et al 1995, Wensing & Van Der Weijden 1998, Yano et al 1995), providing research information alone, management approaches and social influence approaches. Most of the reviews concur with Oxman et al's (1995) assertion that there are 'no magic bullets' when it comes to changing professional practice or attitudes. Based on the evidence, multifaceted approaches to change, whilst more expensive, have the most impact. However, this impact is unpredictable and doesn't always work across every situation.

Specific interventions

A number of systematic reviews examine whether or not specific approaches are useful for clinicians or managers seeking to introduce change. It should be stressed that, in examining these interventions, good-quality evaluative methodology has been weighted above nurse-specific content.

Educational outreach

Academic or educational outreach visits involves trained individuals going out to practice environments to help promote the utilisation of research findings in practice. We have used this approach at York in the area of compression bandaging for venous leg ulceration, but it has proved particularly successful in the prescribing arena. Until now, most of the work has been conducted in North American settings with doctors, but the approach may be useful in attempting to change practice amongst nurses. The effect of outreach approaches is maximised when they are conducted alongside a social marketing framework. The National Research Register (www.update-software.com/NRR/) gives contact details of researchers currently examining the value of educational outreach in the UK and some of these studies are specific to nursing, for example, 'An evaluation of the effectiveness and cost effectiveness of audit and feedback and educational outreach in improving nursing practice and outcomes' and 'Educational outreach in diabetes to encourage practice nurses to respond to guidelines to control hypertension and hyperlipidaemia in primary and shared care (EDEN): a randomised trial using a blocked reciprocal control design'. Generally, 'inter active' approaches to educating groups of professionals may yield positive results (Bero et al 1998). Grimshaw et al's (2004) analysis of educational outreach (both on its own and alongside other strategies) provides an estimate of a 6% improvement in absolute performance. More recently an update of a 1997 systematic review (O'Brien et al 2007) concludes that the effects on prescribing behaviour of educational outreach visits, whilst small, can be significant. However, in terms of other (non-prescribing) behaviour in healthcare professionals, the results vary from small to modest, in ways that cannot be easily explained from the evidence.

Reminders

Reminders, whether manual or electronic, have been shown to be effective in improving preventive care (Shea et al 1996) and general management of patients. Grimshaw et al (2004) suggest that improvements in performance of up to 14% can be possible. However, as nurses increasingly diagnose and treat common conditions (such as asthma), their effect in relation to improving diagnostic behaviour is uncertain (Hunt et al 1998). Additionally, the evidence in favour of reminders as a component of a change strategy is strengthened as evaluations have been derived from a wide range of populations and clinical areas. Perhaps most significant is the work of Fry and Neff (2009) which examines the role of prompts and reminders in a health promotion context (a key part of many nurse's roles). They found that reminders could help enhance the effectiveness of attempts to influence diet, weight loss and exercise. However, as with so many interventions aimed at changing behaviours, their effects were not consistent or entirely predictable – they were, however, broadly positive.

Audit and feedback

It is doubtful that clinical audit, on its own, is a sufficient mechanism for sustained change. Those studies looking at whether audit and feedback approaches to change result in improved behaviours (Balas et al 1996, Buntinx et al 1993, Thomson et al 1999) report at best only moderate improvement. The impact of the technique is greatest when baseline adherence to guidelines is low and when feedback on performance is delivered very intensively (Jamtvedt et al 2006).

Local opinion leaders

Thomson et al (1999) report that local opinion leaders as conduits for change have mixed effects on professional practice. However, we don't always know what local opinion leaders do, and descriptions of their characteristics are often lacking (Doumit et al 2007). Thomson et al (1999) suggest that further research is required to determine the identifying characteristics of leaders and the circumstances in which they are likely to influence the practice of their peers. Bero et al (1998) suggest that colleagues nominated by peers as 'educationally influential' might be a useful characteristic to focus on. Our own work, however, suggests that it is 'clinical credibility' (in the form of experience) rather than research competence or awareness that proves influential in getting nurses to engage with imparted information (Thompson et al 2000). In a multiple case site study, we found that nurses often perceived other nurses as an influential block on them using research. Local opinion leaders (often those embodying the clinical nurse specialist role) were a powerful force for change.

Local consensus approaches

Mulhall and Le May (1999, p. 200) recognise that 'ownership of the [change] project by nurses is important' and this statement is borne out by the evidence. Bero et al (1998) report that inclusion of stakeholder professionals in discussions to ensure their perception of the change problem as 'important' is developed and their response defined as 'appropriate' can exert some effect. However, the results of their scrutiny are mixed and consensus alone should not be relied upon.

Patient-mediated interventions

If a patient asked you to justify your choice of wound dressing or urinary catheter, would it change your approach? This kind of question lies at the core of patient-mediated interventions. Providing information to patients to use in a specific way in professional consultations can, in theory, exert an impact on the behaviour of clinicians. For example, many professionals are increasingly encountering the 'internet-informed' patient and anecdotally, I have encountered healthcare professionals who claim that this 'makes them think twice' about the sorts of information and care provided. However, here too results are mixed and patient-mediated approaches are not a sufficient stand-alone mechanism for cultural shift.

Multifaceted interventions

In general, successful change interventions are multifaceted and targeted to combat specific local contextual factors or barriers to change. The theoretical basis for the combining of interventions is often unclear and results in something akin to a 'kitchen sink' (as in 'everything but the') approach to strategy. This may explain the empirical truth that 'more is not necessarily better' (Grimshaw et al 2004).

Making the most of what is on offer: why 'passive' approaches to change may not be as bad as we think

Those sources of research-based knowledge which many nurses rely on, such as didactic lecture-style study days, passively disseminated clinical practice guidelines, lecture notes, educational videos and protocols, seem to generate only marginal (at best) gains on performance. Freemantle et al (1997), in a review of printed educational materials, found no statistically significant improvements in practice. Similarly, Bero and colleagues (1998) report that didactic-style educational meetings are not useful for inducing change in practice. However, it is clear that whilst gains in performance may only be marginal, the gains in performance for expensive multifaceted interventions may – in absolute terms – not be that much higher, particularly where those interventions are not targeted or lack a strong theoretical foundation. Any strategy must take into account the costs involved. Comprehensive, multifaceted interventions which are ill thought out and expensive may be less useful than passive strategies that are cheaper.

Real-life examples of changing practice and culture

Case 1: A national approach

In the course of teaching nurses about evidence-based health care, the comment is often made that evidence-based health care is only for the 'technical' aspects of nursing or those roles that are seen as 'cutting edge' in nursing and health care (such as the discipline of advanced practitioners). In the UK, however, policy makers and the professions are using a series of national benchmarks alongside audit, education and practice development to apply the principles of evidence-based health care to the basics of essential aspects of patient care in areas such as maintaining privacy and dignity, communication, continence and pressure area care. The policy initiative – called the 'essence of care' – focuses on a series of standards (benchmarks) that are derived from research evidence and adjusted in response to structured consultation with patients, carers and other stakeholders.

The benchmarks are designed to be tailored to local service delivery contexts via the PDSA framework (Plan, Do, Study, and Act), a technique for testing 'change ideas'. Local operationalisation of the benchmarks has exposed the variations between services with respect to their location in the cycle of PDSA. Conversely, the local nature of the operationalisation has resulted in systems that are planned, implemented and evaluated with local context in mind. The national governmental, policy and professional 'steer' has many advantages, some of which are present in the review of the characteristics of innovation offered by Greenhalgh and colleagues (2004).

The standards themselves are evidence based, represent policy concerns and incorporate the values of users and the input of expert clinicians. The nature of the implementation process allows for trialling of the change ideas associated with progress towards the standards. The linkage to local and national audit processes allows for demonstration of progress (or, conversely, the possibility of a lack of it) – a powerful driver in an era of (limited) competition between providers for patients and inter provider comparisons of performance. The standards have high degrees of work relevance and are designed to produce improved and visible task performance. Through the link with audit activity, there is the potential for feedback of task performance and the standards' roles as frameworks for action offer a degree of feed-forward guidance for specific tasks associated with nursing roles. Despite having uniform standards to adhere to, different UK healthcare providers are at different locations in the PDSA cycle.

Changes in the 'culture' of the national workforce are much harder to demonstrate than changes in the activities of individuals or teams charged with implementing this policy. Many of the UK reports on progress towards meeting these standards detail the 'activity' that surrounds the implementation – for example, the establishment of a forum, the appointment of 'champions' and the drafting of best practice. What is less common is the reporting of changes in patient outcome and workforce culture arising from the kind of multifaceted and targeted interventions that develop locally in response to national initiatives such as this. The link between changes in outcome and targeted multifaceted interventions is clearer in Case 2.

Case 2: A co-ordinated approach in the context of high-quality evaluation

Horbar and colleagues (2004) used a cluster randomised clinical trial as an opportunity to evaluate the success of a collaborative multifaceted change intervention to increase the uptake of surfactant (a substance that reduces the surface tension in fragile lungs) in neonatal infants in 57 neonatal intensive care units. The intervention was based around three key components:

- *audit* (1) and *individualised confidential feedback* (2) on peer comparison-related performance regarding administration and timing of surfactant, and delivery room practice for infants of 23–29 weeks' gestation

- a *workshop* (3) made up of didactic sessions, facilitated site team exercises, and multi-institutional group exercises. The intervention was designed to promote four key cultural 'habits' (change, evidence-based practice, systems thinking, and collaborative learning). The sites were all supported via quarterly conference calls and an email discussion list. Control sites simply received centre-specific, confidential performance reports.

The effect of the intervention on routine administration in the delivery room was clinically and statistically significant. The relative benefit increase associated with the intervention was 200% (95% CI 176–228) with 55% of the intervention group (as opposed to 18% of the controls) routinely administering surfactant. The study failed to detect changes in mortality (it was not designed to do so), but does illustrate that theoretically informed multifaceted interventions can exert a powerful effect on the processes of healthcare delivery – processes that are influenced (and maintained) by the culture of the organisation.

Change as a result of attempts at specifically influencing culture is often characterised by a series of decidedly non-linear periods of growth, plateaus, apparent demise and re-emergence: it is transformational (Illes & Sutherland 2001) (see Fig. 10.2).

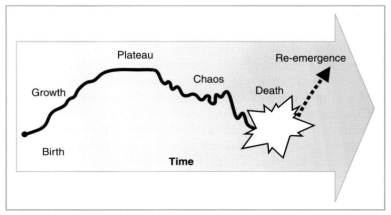

Figure 10.2 Transformational organisational change (derived from Illes & Sutherland 2001)

Case 3: The mediating effects of transformational change and local context

Newman et al (2000) developed a theoretically informed, locally tailored, multifaceted intervention explicitly designed to change the prevailing culture of practice. The developers used a combination of specific change interventions ('link nurses', clinical supervision and educational outreach) nested within a broader action research framework. Perhaps crucially, they chose not to inject extra resources to support the change intervention, ostensibly to increase its 'realism'. They chose problems that were raised by the ward staff involved, and used the generic evidence-based skills and techniques of question formulation, searching, appraisal, changing practice and evaluation to address them. Changes in culture and processes of healthcare delivery were measured using a combination of indicators such as staff sickness (believed to be linked to morale), patient complaints, the numbers of PICO questions generated (see Chapter 2) and searches undertaken, the nurses' perception of the impact of the project, and the quality of nursing documentation.

The strategic intervention met with only partial success. On the positive side, the project resulted in a number of improvements in work role and design (introduction of team and named nurses, better patient assessment, a standardised format for handing over patients – with accompanying clinical questions – team and self-duty-rostering and performance review). The strategy also reduced sickness by 10 days per month (95% CI 5.3–14.3) and was perceived as enhancing communication, confidence, leadership and teamwork. On the less positive side, however, many of the organisational changes were not sustained, systems to link question formulation and searching failed to be fully operationalised; some nursing cultural subgroups actively resisted the project and the ward manager served as a negative role model for evidence-based practice. In the words of the researchers, 'changes were fragile and easily reversed'.

The evaluation took place over 10 months and what was observed may only have captured a small element of the transformational change sequence. The absence of extra resources – if only as a marker of organisational commitment and 'buy-in' – was possibly also a contributory factor to the intervention's relatively small long-term impact. Ultimately, the project leaders concluded that clinical units are unlikely to operationalise evidence-based practice without considering local professional and organisational contexts. As well as local contexts, they highlight particular structural issues such as the priority afforded to evidence-based practice by organisations; the matching of resources to workloads; preparing clinical leaders and nurses for using evidence-based practice skills and deploying new knowledge; and the need for ongoing development of 'generic' critical thinking and problem-solving skills (Newman et al 2000).

This last example represents a caveat for those considering trying to change organisational culture. Even with diagnosis, a theoretical framework and a multi-approach strategy using validated techniques, the results are often far from certain and nothing can be assumed.

This example from the King's Fund report *Getting Better with Evidence* (Wye & McClenahan 2000) suggests that sustainable change is possible with attention to the kinds of local, contextual and structural issues highlighted by Newman and colleagues.

Case 4: Primary care leg ulcer clinics

In this example, a group of inner-city tissue viability specialist nurses (TVNs) wanted to develop, implement and audit their local guidelines on managing leg ulcers and then go on to set up two community-based leg ulcer clinics. The aim of this was to reduce variations in practice and outcomes across the trust and to reduce inappropriate referrals to an already busy complex wound clinic.

The nurses developed a fivefold strategy:

- *Locally developed guidelines*: based on an inclusive, multidisciplinary development process that was actively 'marketed' in trust settings at lunch times

- *Opinion leaders*: the two well-respected TVNs worked with nurses on a part-time basis and ensured that they also worked with consultants and local GPs
- *Educational workshops*: these took place 'in-service' and were aimed at familiarising nurses with the guidelines and, crucially, learning to relate the guidelines to real patients and patient problems
- *Targeted meetings and multidisciplinary training*: these focused on generating sufficient interest in practitioners so that they wanted to host clinics. Moreover, these involved targeting the most enthusiastic practitioner in a local team in order that they would persuade their more sceptical colleagues
- *Training and feedback*: the TVNs visited each clinic once a month and offered real-time training, support and, crucially, the application of the guidelines during patient consultations.

This approach has led to the development of two clinics, with a third in progress, with broad cross-disciplinary support for the new ways of working. However, the team failed to collect patient data before or after the development of the clinics, which meant they had no baseline criteria for measuring their success. As well as this design fault, the team had to struggle against the very real constraints of underfunding, recruitment difficulties, competing priorities and variable morale and enthusiasm amongst staff. The qualitative comments of staff reveal that relatively small changes, such as changing the ways in which clinical nurse specialists work (giving them a trust-wide remit with responsibility for individual training and professional development), can yield good results, even in the context of a far from perfect strategy: 'Having (the clinical nurse specialist) there to discuss different things makes a difference. When you are seeing seven leg ulcers in a row, it leads to better practice. We are using the leg ulcer care programme lots...the professional development is the best part of it'.

So a relatively small change can have a significant impact on the development of others' expertise and professional development. Importantly, the team involved learned from their mistakes and were trying to factor in the solutions for the future: 'We would invest a proportion of the project's resources in a baseline audit because demonstrating improvement in healing rates provides the ultimate proof that an initiative to upgrade the care of patients with leg ulcers is working'.

Ultimately, the researchers conclude that the team's greatest (cultural) achievement was their contribution to the replacement of '...a severely fragmented, demoralised organisation with one where staff are enthusiastic and open to learning'.

Case 5: EBP and the importance of context in two US hospitals

Stetler and colleagues (Stetler et al 2009) describe two hospitals in the United States (one 350 bed academic medical centre and one 400 bed community unit) at very different stages of adoption of evidence based practice. The academic medical centre was perceived as being three-quarters of the way toward fully integrating EBP into its daily work, whilst the more rural case was only one-fifth of the way toward full integration. The academic centre was classed as a 'role model' for integrated EBP, with the rural hospital classed as a 'beginner' in terms of progress toward full integration. When the lessons learned from the stories of implementing a culture change in the two sites were pulled together it was clear that issues of strategy (clear, strong and consistently applied), leadership (strong, visible and championed by executives who think proactively), but above all targeting of interventions at contextual barriers and a general sense of active management of the 'how' (will we change?) as well as the 'what' (will we change?) varied. The result was that leadership, organisational learning capacity, and research utilisation were all higher in the hospital that had paid most attention to an integrated and strategic approach to dealing with contextual factors as they developed over time.

Conclusion: culture, practice change and evidence-based health care

This chapter has shown how complex an entity organisational culture is and how difficult it is to try and mould something that is contingent on so many other factors. Despite this complexity,

I have outlined a number of strategies which, if used in conjunction with broad and specific interventions, could reasonably be expected to yield some results.

Most people would agree that evidence-based health care should be a reality, but very often tips on how to deliver the necessary behavioural (and, by implication, cultural) changes are lacking. This chapter has argued that strategy and working with proven approaches can help add the local detail necessary to complement the national directives.

As Oxman et al (1995) point out, there are 'no magic bullets' when attempting organisational change. However, by strategically arming yourself with a number of different techniques for changing culture and behaviour, you can at least give yourself and your team a fighting chance of successfully introducing change.

To conclude, the clinician or manager considering change should employ a good diagnostic work-up of the factors likely to hinder or promote research use in decisions. This should focus on the levels of individuals, teams and the organisation and consider strategically targeting barriers and subgroups within each of these elements. Moreover, initial efforts should focus on those areas over which the team has a modicum of control (for example, the text-based ward resources amassed by the ward, unit or practice; the roles of key individuals such as the clinical nurse specialist or the link nurse; or the support and nature of skills training). Whilst being aware of the likely time scale involved and the non-linear progress of change, ensure that the process is seen as cyclical, with audit and feedback designed into the strategy.

References

Allen, D., Gillen, E., Rixson, L., 2009. The Effectiveness of Integrated Care Pathways for Adults and Children in Health Care Settings: A Systematic Review. Joanna Briggs Library of Systematic Reviews 7 (3), 80–129. Available online at http://www.joannabriggs.edu.au/pdf/SRLib_2009_7_3.pdf. Accessed 7th September 2010.

Balas, E.A., Austin, S.M., Mitchell, J., et al., 1996. The clinical value of computerized information services: a review of 98 randomised clinical trials. Arch. Fam. Med. 5, 271–278.

Beaudry, J.S., 1989. The effectiveness of continuing medical education: a quantitative synthesis. J. Contin. Educ. Health Prof. 9, 285–307.

Bero, L.A., Grilli, R., Grimshaw, J.M., et al., 1998. Closing the gap between research and practice: an overview of systematic reviews of interventions to promote the implementation of research findings. Br. Med. J. 317, 465–468.

Bertram, D.A., Brooks-Bertram, P.A., 1977. The evaluation of continuing medical education: a literature review. Health. Educ. Monogr. 5, 330–362.

Brown, S.J., 1999. Knowledge for health care practice: a guide to using research evidence. W B Saunders, London.

Buntinx, F., Winkens, R., Grol, R., et al., 1993. Influencing diagnostic and preventative performance in ambulatory care by feedback and reminders. A review. Fam. Pract. 10, 219–228.

Cameron, G., Wren, A.M., 1999. Reconstructing organisational culture: a process using multiple perspectives. Public Health Nurs. 16 (2), 96–101.

Covell, D.G., Gwen, C., Uman, R.N., Manning, P.R., 1985. Information needs in office practice: are they being met? Ann. Intern. Med. 103, 596–599.

Davies, H.T.O., Nutley, S.M., Mannion, R., 2000. Organisational culture and quality of health care. Qual. Health Care 9, 111–119.

Davis, D.A., Thomson, M.A., Oxman, A.D., et al., 1995. Changing physician performance: a systematic review of the effect of continuing medical education strategies. J. Am. Med. Assoc. 274, 700–705.

Department of Health, 2007. World class commissioning: Vision. HMSO, London.

DiCenso, A., Cullum, N., Ciliska, D., 1998. Implementation forum. Implementing evidence-based nursing: some misconceptions. Evid. Based Nurs. 1 (2), 38–40.

DiCenso, A., Bayley, L., Haynes, R.B., 2009. EBN Notebook: Accessing pre-appraised evidence: fine-tuning the 5S model into a 6S model. Evid. Based Nurs. 12 (4), 99–101.

Doumit, G., Gattellari, M., Grimshaw, J., O'Brien, M.A., 2007. Local opinion leaders: effects on professional practice and health care outcomes. Cochrane Database Syst. Rev. 2007 (4) Art. No.: CD000125. doi:10.1002/14651858.CD000125.pub3.

Ferlie, E.J., Gabbay, L., Fitzgerald, L.E., Dopson, S., 2001. Evidence-based medicine and organisational change. In: Ashburner, L. (Ed.), Organisational behaviour and organisational studies in health care: reflections on the future. Palgrave, Basingstoke.

Freemantle, N., Harvey, E., Wolf, F., Grimshaw, J., Grilli, R., Bero, L., 1997. Printed educational materials: effects on professional practice and health care outcomes. Cochrane Database of Systematic Reviews. Issue 2. Art. No.: CD000172. DOI: 10.1002/14651858.CD000172.

Fry, J., Neff, R., 2009. Periodic prompts and reminders in health promotion and health behavior interventions: systematic review. J. Med. Internet Res. 11 (2), e16.

Funk, S., Champagne, M.T., Wiese, R.A., Tornquist, E.M., 1991. Barriers: the Barriers to Research Utilization Scale. Appl. Nurs. Res. 4 (1), 39–45.

Greenhalgh, T., Glenn, R., Bate, P., et al., 2004. Diffusion of innovations in service organisations: systematic review and recommendations. Millbank Q. 82 (4), 581–629.

Grimshaw, J.M., Thomas, R.E., MacLennan, G., et al., 2004. Effectiveness and efficiency of guideline dissemination and implementation strategies. Health Technol. Assess. 8 (6), i–iv, 1–72.

Grol, R., 1992. Implementing guidelines in general practice care. Qual. Health Care 1, 184–191.

Haynes, R.B., 2001. Of studies, syntheses, synopses, and systems: the '4S' evolution of services for finding current best evidence. ACP J. Club 134, A11–A13.

Horbar, J.D., Carpenter, J.H., Buzas, J., et al., 2004. Collaborative quality improvement to promote evidence-based surfactant for preterm infants: a cluster randomised trial. Br. Med. J. 329, 1004.

Hunt, D.L., Haynes, R.B., Hanna, S.E., et al., 1998. Effects of computer based decision support on physician performance and patient outcomes. A systematic review. J. Am. Med. Assoc. 280, 1339–1346.

Illes, V., Sutherland, K., 2001. Organisational change: a review for health care managers, professionals and researchers. NCC SDO, London.

Jamtvedt, G., Young, J.M., Kristoffersen, D.T., O'Brien, M.A., Oxman, A.D., 2006. Audit and feedback: effects on professional practice and health care outcomes. Cochrane Database Syst. Rev. (2). Art. No.: CD000259. doi:10.1002/14651858.CD000259.pub2.

Lloyd, J.S., Abrahamson, S., 1979. Effectiveness of continuing medical education: a review of the evidence. Eval. Health Prof. 2, 251–280.

McCaughan, D., Thompson, C., Cullum, N., Sheldon, T.A., Raynor, P., 2005. Nurse practitioner and practice nurses' use of research information in clinical decision making: findings from an exploratory study. Fam. Pract. 22 (5), 490–497.

Muir Gray, J.A., 1997. Evidence-based health care: how to make health policy and management decisions. Churchill Livingstone, Edinburgh.

Mulhall, A., Le May, A., 1999. Nursing research: dissemination and implementation. Churchill Livingstone, London.

Newman, M., Papadopoulos, I., Melifonwu, R., 2000. Developing organisational systems and culture to support evidence-based practice: the experience of the Evidence-based Ward Project. Evid. Based Nurs. 3, 103–105.

NHS Centre for Reviews and Dissemination (CRD), 1999. Getting evidence into practice. Effective Health Care Bulletin 5 (1), 1–16.

NHS Executive, 1999. Clinical effectiveness: what it's all about. Available online at: www.doh.gov.uk/pub/docs/doh/aep.pdf. Accessed 7th September 2010.

O'Brien, M.A., Rogers, S., Jamtvedt, G., et al., 2007. Educational outreach visits: effects on professional practice and health care outcomes. Cochrane Database Syst. Rev. (4) Art. No.: CD000409. doi:10.1002/14651858.CD000409.pub2.

Oxman, A., Thomson, M.A., Davis, D.A., Haynes, R.B., 1995. No magic bullets: a systematic review of 102 trials of interventions to improve professional practice. Can. Med. Assoc. J. 153 (10), 1423–1431.

Parker, M., 2000. Organisational culture and identity: unity and division at work. Sage, London.

Sackett, D.L., Strauss, S.E., Richardson, W.S., Rosenberg, W., Haynes, R.B., 2000. Evidence-based medicine: how to practise and teach EBM. Churchill Livingstone, London.

Schon, D., 1983. The reflective practitioner: how professionals think in action. Basic Books, New York.

Scott, T., Mannion, R., Davies, H.T.O., Marshall, M., 2003. Implementing culture change in health care: theory and practice. Int. J. Qual. Health Care 15 (2), 111–118.

Secretary of State for Health, 1998. A first class service: quality in the new NHS. Department of Health, London.

Secretary of State for Health, 2000. The NHS plan. Department of Health, London.

Shea, S., DuMouchel, W., Bahamonde, L., 1996. A meta-analysis of 16 randomised controlled trials to evaluate computer-based clinical reminder systems for preventative care in the ambulatory setting. J. Am. Med. Inform. Assoc. 3, 399–409.

Stetler, C., Ritchie, J., Rycroft-Malone, J., Schultz, A.A., Charns, M.P., 2009. Institutionalizing evidence-based practice: an organizational case study using a model of strategic change. Implementation Science 4 (1), 78.

Thomas, LH., Cullum, NA., McColl, E., Rousseau, N., Soutter, J., Steen, N., 1999. Guidelines in professions allied to medicine. Cochrane Database of Systematic Reviews. Issue 1. Art. No.: CD000349. DOI: 10.1002/14651858.CD000349.

Thompson, C., McCaughan, D., Cullum, N., Sheldon, T.A., Thompson, D.R., Mulhall, A., 2000. Nurses' use of research information in clinical decision making: a descriptive and analytical study – final report. NHS R&D, NCC SDO, London.

Thomson, M.A., Oxman, A.D., Davis, D.A., Haynes, R.B., Freemantle, N., Harvey, E.L., 1999. Outreach visits to improve health professional practice and health care outcomes (Cochrane Review). Cochrane Library (1). Update Software, Oxford.

Waddell, D.L., 1991. The effects of continuing education on nursing practice: a meta-analysis. J. Contin. Educ. Nurs. 22, 113–118.

Wensing, M., Van Der Weijden, T.R.G., 1998. Implementing guidelines and innovations in general practice: which interventions are effective? Br. J. Gen. Pract. 48, 991–997.

Wye, L., McClenahan, J., 2000. Getting better with evidence: experiences of putting evidence into practice. King's Fund, London.

Yano, E.M., Fink, A., Hirsch, S.H., et al., 1995. Helping practices reach primary care goals. Lessons from the literature. Arch. Intern. Med. 155, 1146–1156.

Glossary

Absolute risk reduction (ARR) and increase (ARI) This figure tells us the size of the difference between outcomes in the intervention (or exposure) group and outcomes in the control group. It is the absolute arithmetical difference between the experimental (or exposure) event rate (EER) and the control event rate (CER). To calculate: [EER − CER].

Action research Investigators and participants collaborate to improve a social situation through change interventions. The emphasis is on professional development and empowerment of participants.

Allocation concealment Ensuring that the person who enrols individuals into a study is unaware of the group to which that individual will be allocated. Techniques include using sequentially numbered, sealed, opaque envelopes, with each envelope containing details of the group to which that individual is to be allocated (e.g. group A or group B). Central randomisation services are also used, where people not involved in the study hold the randomisation details. At the time of allocating the individual to a group, the investigator contacts the service to find out whether that individual is to go into group A or group B.

Bias Systematic error in the design, conduct or interpretation of a study that may distort the results of the study away from the 'truth'.

Blinding (masking) Concealing whether or not the participant is receiving (or has received) the experimental intervention. In an ideal study, the research participant, the people administering the intervention(s), the people assessing the outcomes and the data analysts will be blinded. The terms single-blind, double-blind or triple-blind are sometimes used to indicate the level of blinding. For example, where both the participants and the investigators assessing the outcomes are blinded, the trial may be classified as double-blind. However, it is important to note that these terms are not used consistently.

Boolean operators Used when searching electronic databases to combine search terms. They include AND, OR and NOT.

Case control study An observational study where a group of individuals with the target disorder (cases) and a group of individuals without the target disorder (controls) are identified. Researchers look back in time to try and identify whether the exposure of interest was more prevalent in one group than the other.

Case study An in-depth investigation of an individual person, group of people, organisation or event using a variety of sources of data.

Case series A study reporting on a series of patients who have all experienced an outcome of interest, and where there is no control group.

CATs & CATmaker software CAT is the abbreviated term for critically appraised topic. It is a summary of individual item(s) of evidence that you create yourself in response to an information need. The Centre for Evidence-Based Medicine produces CATmaker software which can be used to create CATs and which includes a facility to calculate figures such as the number needed to treat, etc.

Clinical effectiveness This term is used in two ways: first, as shorthand for the processes used to improve the quality of health care; second, to refer to the extent to which a specific clinical intervention, when deployed in the field for a particular patient or population, delivers the intended outcomes such that the benefits outweigh the harms.

Clinical governance A framework through which healthcare organisations are accountable for continuously improving the quality of health services and safeguarding high standards of care.

Cohort study An observational study where patients exposed to a drug or other agent are identified and followed forward in time to see whether they develop particular outcomes. People not exposed to the agent (i.e. a control group) may be included in the study.

Confidence interval (CI) Research studies use samples from the population. If the same study was carried out 100 times on different samples of the same population, 100 different results would be obtained. These results would spread around a true but unknown value. The confidence interval estimates this sampling variation. Thus we can think of the confidence interval as the range within which it is probable that the population value lies. It is possible to calculate this range from the data obtained in a single study. By convention, the 95% confidence interval is often used, i.e. the true population value will lie between the specified range in 95% of cases. For example, if a study reported a difference in mortality rates between two groups as 10% with an upper 95% CI limit of 13% and lower 95% confidence limit of 7%, we know that in 95% of cases the true mortality difference, for the population, is between 7% and 13%.

Confirmability The extent to which research findings are determined by participants rather than by the perspectives or motives of the researcher.

Confounder A factor that affects the observed relationship between the variables under investigation.

Constant comparative analysis Used in qualitative studies, the researcher constantly seeks out cases in the dataset during the collection of the data that support or 'shape' provisional hypotheses.

Control event rate (CER) This is the proportion of individuals in the control group in whom the outcome (event) is observed.

Control group The control group in a study is that group of individuals who do not receive the intervention or exposure, or who receive a placebo. Their outcomes are compared with those of the intervention group (the group receiving the intervention or exposure). They serve to 'control' for whether the patients in the intervention group would have improved or deteriorated regardless of the intervention or exposure.

Credibility The extent to which findings are believable.

Critical appraisal The process of systematically evaluating a piece of evidence in terms of validity (i.e. the extent to which the results may be affected by bias), findings (i.e. interpreting the results) and applicability (i.e. the extent to which the findings may be applicable to your own clinical setting/patients).

Cross-sectional study Data are collected from a representative sample of individuals at the same point in time.

Dependability Used in qualitative research, the extent to which research findings are repeatable if the research is repeated in the same or similar participants or context.

Ethnography The nature of organisations, culture or communities in their native settings.

Experimental event rate (EER) The proportion of participants in the treatment (intervention) group in whom the outcome (event) is observed.

Grounded theory Development of new theoretical perspectives based on (grounded in) people's lived experiences.

Incidence The number of new cases of a disease occurring in the population at risk, in a specified period of time.

Intention-to-treat analysis Study participants are analysed in the groups to which they were randomised even if they did not receive the planned intervention or if they deviated from the study protocol. Intention-to-treat analysis mimics real-life situations because it investigates the outcomes following a management decision to use a particular treatment.

Inter-rater (or inter-observer) reliability Measures the extent to which an instrument or test gives consistent results when applied by different investigators under exactly the same circumstances and where the variable being measured remains unchanged.

Intra-rater (or intra-observer) reliability Measures the extent to which an instrument or test gives consistent results when applied by the same investigator at two or more time points under exactly the same circumstances and where the variable being measured remains unchanged.

Kappa coefficient (κ) A statistical test used to indicate the extent of agreement between observers' measurements, adjusted for the amount of agreement that could be expected due to chance alone. The results are reported between 0 and 1. The nearer the result is to 1, the better the agreement between the observers' measurements.

Likelihood ratio See negative and positive likelihood ratios.

Median The midpoint on a scale. Half of the observations have a value less than or equal to the median and half have a value greater than or equal to the median.

Member (respondent) checking Used in qualitative research, the process of feeding back the researcher's interpretations of the data to informants (the people involved in generating the data) to determine whether they recognise and agree with them.

Meta-analysis Used in systematic reviews, this is the process of statistically combining the results from a number of studies. Meta-analysis is not appropriate in all systematic reviews.

Narrative enquiry Exploring the lives of individuals through their narratives or stories.

Naturalistic enquiry Relating to qualitative research, phenomena are studied within their natural setting rather than within a superficial or controlled one. The approach aims to minimise investigator manipulation of the study setting and places no prior constraint on what the outcomes will be.

Negative case analysis Used in qualitative research, the process of actively searching for cases that appear to be inconsistent with the emerging analysis.

Negative likelihood ratio The ratio of true-negative results to false-negative results. A negative likelihood ratio of 0.5 means that a negative test result is half as likely to occur in patients with the condition as in patients without the condition.

Negative predictive value The proportion of people with negative test results who do not have the target disorder (should be high).

Number needed to harm The number of patients to receive the intervention for one additional person to experience an episode of harm, over a specified period of time. To calculate: 1/ARR.

Number needed to treat The number of patients that need to be treated if a beneficial outcome is to occur in one additional person. To calculate: 1/ARR.

Odds The probability of an event happening, i.e. the ratio of the number of people having the outcome of interest to the number of people not having the outcome of interest.

Odds ratio The ratio of the odds of an event in the treatment (or exposure) group compared to the odds of the event in the control (or unexposed) group.

Ontology Relates to the nature of things within the world: the assumptions and beliefs we hold about how the world is made up.

Phenomenology Relates to the nature of individuals' personal experiences.

Placebo In the context of a placebo-controlled clinical trial, this is a biologically inert substance given to participants in the control arm of a trial. The placebo is similar in every other way to the biologically active intervention administered to participants in the treatment arm of the trial. It is used to conceal which arm of the trial the participants are in.

Positive likelihood ratio The ratio of true-positive results to false-positive results. A positive likelihood ratio of 8.5 means that a positive test result is 8.5 times as likely to occur in patients with the condition as in patients without the condition. (A positive likelihood ratio of 1 means that a positive test is equally as likely to occur in patients with the condition as in patients without the condition.)

Positive predictive value The proportion of people with positive test results who have the target disorder (should be high).

Prevalence This is the number of cases of the outcome of interest (e.g. a disease) in a defined population at a given point in time.

Quantitative research Seeks to describe phenomena through measuring and quantifying the relationship between the variables or characteristics being studied.

Qualitative research Seeks to describe phenomena through the meanings, experiences, practices and views of individuals within their natural settings. Qualitative research aims to understand real-world situations as they unfold, from the point of view of the people who live in these worlds.

Random allocation Individuals participating in the trial have a defined probability (usually 50%, i.e. an equal chance) of being allocated to either the intervention or the control group. Computer packages or printed random number tables are usually used to generate a list of random numbers (i.e. numbers with no discernable sequence or order) which indicate the group to which each individual is to be randomised. So, for example, even numbers might indicate allocation to the intervention group and odd numbers to the control group. The group to which each individual is to be allocated is not predictable.

Randomised controlled trial (RCT) A study in which individuals are assigned to the experimental intervention group or to the comparison group(s) by random allocation.

Reflexivity A technique used in qualitative research, especially in the analysis of data, where the author reflects on how she or he may have shaped or influenced the research findings.

Relative benefit increase (RBI) The proportional increase in rates of beneficial events between the experimental and control group. To calculate: [EER – CER]/CER.

Relative risk (RR) The ratio of the risk in one group compared to the other.

Relative risk increase (RRI) The proportional increase in rates of harmful or undesirable events between the experimental and control group. To calculate: [EER – CER]/CER.

Relative risk reduction (RRR) The proportional reduction in rates of harmful or undesirable events between the experimental and control group. To calculate: [EER – CER]/CER.

Reliability See inter-rater and intra-rater reliability.

Sample Research is carried out on a subgroup of the population. This subgroup is often referred to as the study sample. A variety of sampling methods can be employed to select the sample depending on the purpose of the research.

Sensitivity When applied to diagnostic tests, sensitivity refers to the proportion of people with a target disorder who have a positive test result.

Specificity When applied to diagnostic tests, specificity refers to the proportion of people who do not have a target disorder who have a negative test result.

Statistical significance The likelihood of a result occurring by chance. By convention, the level at which a result is said to be statistically significant is set at 5%, i.e. when there is less than a 5% probability that the result happened by chance, it is said to be statistically significant. This is usually written in the form of $P \leq 0.05$. The P value does not, however, tell us how clinically important the result is.

Systematic review A summary of research evidence pertinent to a specified question in which systematic and explicit methods are used to identify, select, critically appraise and synthesise the available research evidence. Systematic reviews are research studies in their own right and are sometimes called 'secondary research'.

Thick description A term used in qualitative research. A very detailed account of the methodological and interpretive strategy in the form of fieldnotes.

Transferability The extent to which research findings are transferable, from the context within which the research study was undertaken to another.

Triangulation The phenomenon under investigation is examined from different perspectives using two or more methods (or data sources/data sources/theories/investigators). Findings of the different methods are cross checked and interpreted against each other.

Truncation Used in searching electronic databases, truncation ensures that all terms that have the same text stem are found. For example, a search for the truncated word 'child' will retrieve articles containing the terms child, childhood, childless, children, etc. The truncation symbol varies according to the database provider. Examples of symbols are the asterisk (child*), dollar sign (child$) or % sign (child%).

Wildcard Used in searching electronic databases, a wildcard is a character (in some databases it is a ?) that can be used to replace one or more characters within a word so that articles will be retrieved regardless of the way in which the word is spelt. For example, if the term 'p?ediatric' is searched, articles using the American spelling (pediatric) and articles using the British spelling (paediatric) will be retrieved.

Index

Notes: Page numbers followed by *b* indicates boxes, *f* indicates figures and *t* indicates tables.

Page numbers in **bold** refer to terms in the Glossary